James Adams has taught psychology, sociology and the philosophy of religion in a sixth form centre for over twenty years. He is also the author of *Attached to Coventry City*.

Your work was found to be an informative and thought-provoking read that is sure to appeal to a wide audience. The reader would find much to stimulate them, allowing reflection and understanding to continue in earnest at some distance past the final page. The Board was keen to comment on your dynamic and accessible writing style and how this works to deliver an enhanced appeal to readers... Therefore, we very much feel your work deserves to be published and given the opportunity to be launched for the reading public.

—Austin Macauley Publishers

*

James Adams has been following Coventry City for many years and he is undoubtedly passionate about his team. Coming from the same generation as James, I understand that passion. His memories of growing up in Coventry and following our beloved team make for an enjoyable read.

—Jim Brown: Official historian for Coventry City F.C.

With respect and gratitude for

the pioneering work of John Bowlby and Mary Ainsworth,

the founders of Attachment theory.

James Adams

PASSIONATE

The Psychology of a Passionate Life

To Fiona,
with best wishes
James Adams

AUSTIN MACAULEY PUBLISHERS™

LONDON • CAMBRIDGE • NEW YORK • SHARJAH

A CIP catalogue record for this title is available from the British Library.

ISBN 9781398401693 (Paperback)
ISBN 9781398401709 (ePub e-book)

www.austinmacauley.com

First Published 2022
Austin Macauley Publishers Ltd®
1 Canada Square
Canary Wharf
London
E14 5AA

Acknowledgements

Many thanks to Kathy for editing and improving my English on every page and also to Alan, James and Lana for their unwavering support. Thanks also to Prof. Jeremy Holmes for his positive endorsement, and to the team at Austin Macauley for their initial positivity and oversight of the publication process.

Last, but by no means least, my thanks to those hundreds of students, who have discussed and debated so many ideas and issues with me—always with open, enquiring minds, kind hearts and good humour.

Table of Contents

A life of passion, attachments, crises—and therapy.
And a journey towards positive mental health.

Having been a passionate football supporter and then an enthusiastic convert to evangelical Christianity, James Adams finds his life falling apart in his mid-thirties. Having given up football for his new-found faith and ministry, he eventually loses all his religious beliefs and identity along with his career, a long-term relationship and most of his friends.

In despair, he enters therapy, hoping for a quick fix that will get his life back on track. Instead, he finds a pattern repeating itself: a pattern of passion and loss and the need for further therapy. In his quest to make sense of his chaotic life, he eventually discovers Attachment theory, which becomes the cornerstone of his therapeutic journey—and beyond. But first, in order to be healed in the present, he has to step back into his past—a past he would rather forget.

"The thing about you,
is that you never do anything by halves.
Whatever you do,
you're always passionate about it."
—a friend

Disclaimer

To protect the anonymity of the people mentioned in this book, the names of all have been changed (except those known in the public arena), along with certain geographical locations, chronological sequencing and identifying characteristics.

Introduction

" James, I think you will find that if you want to move forwards, you will first have to look backwards." Those were some of my counsellor's first words, when I started in therapy some three decades ago. They were the last words I wanted to hear. I wanted her to rescue me from my agony now. I wanted a quick fix.

In today's culture of the mass media and social media we are more aware than ever of the mental health problems for people of all ages, with both the government and the younger Royals pitching in with their concern and support. A myriad of therapists and therapies are available to help people of all ages and from all walks of life deal with their perturbing and sometimes frightening problems. For some, a short course of Cognitive Behavioural Therapy or a prescribed medication may help provide some stability and the chance to think clearly to reassess the issues that trouble them. But for many, it may be necessary to 'look backwards' first, to uncover the shaky foundations upon which one's life has been built. In my case, I was well into middle age before I discovered the reasons why my life had become such a chaotic mess. My hope is that others are able to make such important discoveries at a much younger age.

This book is written for anyone who feels a shadow hanging over their life, and who is prepared to dip into their past in order to understand their present and feel more positively about the future. This understanding will be provided by the well-established Life Course psychology in general, and an understanding of Attachment theory in particular, as I have applied both to my own life. Both psychological analysis and some pointers towards positive mental health will be reserved for the final (tenth) section of each chapter, with the roller-coaster narrative taking up the preceding nine sections. It is a story of passion and strange attachments, breakdowns and crises—and a long, slow, recovery. It is not a story of a quick fix, despite several 'AHA!' moments joyously experienced along the way. I hope that for you, the reader, it will bring a greater awareness, even enlightenment, about the roots of your own life. For with awareness comes acceptance, and with acceptance comes the possibility of healing.

In the chapters that follow there are three key words that need some prior clarification:

Passionate is normally understood in relation to a positive, romantic or sexual encounter, although to be passionate about an interest, hobby or sports team is not an uncommon usage. What is less well known is that the root of 'passion' is the Latin passio, 'I suffer'—as in 'the passion of Christ', a 'Passion Play' or 'compassion'—to suffer with or alongside someone. For when people fall passionately in love, they also suffer, for example from separation-anxiety when apart from their beloved. Therefore the title of this book has a double-meaning, and deliberately so. It is a book about the sufferings of passion as well as its pleasures.

Crisis is normally understood in the negative sense of something going seriously wrong, perhaps unexpectedly or dramatically. There are certainly examples of that in the story that follows. However, the root of crisis is the Greek krisis—'a decisive moment', from krino to decide or judge. Therefore a 'crisis' can also be a neutral (or even positive) decision, judgement or event. It is in this broader sense that I use the word in several chapter titles—for within each chapter, you will find crises of many varieties. And of course, some crises that at first seem entirely negative may be viewed later in a more positive light, and vice-versa.

Attachment also has various meanings, with two being relevant for the pages that follow. The word is frequently used in a general sense such as 'I'm very attached to my old record collection'. It also has a specific psychological meaning of: 'a life-affecting emotional bond with a key figure, usually (though not exclusively) a parent or a carer'. It is in this latter psychological sense that I use the term in this book. On the few occasions that I need to express the more general meaning, I shall choose another word or term, so as to avoid confusion. Within the psychological meaning of 'attachment', there are a plethora of related terms, for example 'secure attachment' and these will be explained in the text as the story and analysis proceed.

At the end of the book there are some concluding thoughts about positive mental health, and two personality exercises that have worked well for hundreds of students in the school where I taught. If you feel so inclined, have a go. At the very least they will set you thinking, and possibly re-thinking your life.

Desolation Row
Christmas Eve 1986

I watch in stunned disbelief as Francesca collects her bags, throws them on the backseat of her red VW Golf, then returns to me. She hugs me warmly and at length, before eventually pulling away. She plants a kiss on my forehead—and then she's off. No words were spoken, nor needed, as we had already said it all. A year after her husband had left her, he was coming back from the oil fields in the hope of rekindling their marriage, and she felt she owed him that. For me, however, these last six months had been the most joyous, glorious and wonderful ones of my life, far surpassing anything that football, religion or a long-term relationship had provided.

I watch her car turn the corner for the last time, as she sets out to rebuild her life. But I'm entirely desolate. Incomprehensive, inconsolable and numb. As I stare down my godforsaken street, I realise that it reflects my world within, now that Francesca has gone.

*

It's a dead-end street where I live—and I live at the dead end. Not a suburban cul-de-sac—just a ten-foot wall of old red bricks and breeze blocks, topped off with shards of broken glass in concrete and rusting barbed wire. This is where my street ends—it's my very own Berlin Wall, except there's no Checkpoint Charlie here, just the dim and dingy 'Crown' pub on the corner with its weak Christmas lights and bleak, faded posters. Either side of the street are two rows of back-to-backs, standing tall and creating dark shadows in the bright morning sun. Half of them are boarded up and, on my side, small front yards assault the eyes with their dirty mattresses, burned-out cars and upturned supermarket trolleys. Two large stray dogs scavenge the open bins and chase each other around—and I recall some lines of T. S. Eliot from a happier teenage world, long since left behind:

> *Let us go, through certain half-deserted streets,*
> *The muttering retreats*
> *Of restless nights in one-night cheap hotels* [1]

To other residents, of course, all this may be home—and I do have a house at the dead end. But I'm in shock and scarcely able to move between the Berlin Wall and the burned-out cars. In any case, what possible reason do I have for moving? Where can I possibly go—when both body and soul are stuck at the dead end of Desolation Row?

*

My desolation has been very traumatic and is now complete. Within the past year, I've lost my religious faith and identity, a good career, a long-term relationship and virtually all of my friends—only one remained true. I've now lost Francesca, the most caring and lovely lady who knew me through and through. But most of all, I've lost any sense of who I am—whereas once I thought I knew.

It's now mid-day and I'm still standing here in my front yard, rooted to the spot but rootless, as I peer down the sunlit street asking myself questions to which I have no answers, with a heart breaking with grief over a lost love who I know will not return.

Then suddenly, I have an idea:

> *Oh, do not ask, 'What is it?'*
> *Let us go and make our visit.* [2]

It's a night-time visit to a Midlands town in the grip of an icy blast, for in order to understand my present, I need to revisit my past.

Chapter 1 ~ Childhood Attachments
1951–66

1. The Unforgettable Night
A Midlands town Midnight, January 1951

"It's the police! Open up! It's the police! Open the door!"

Dad grabs his dressing gown and makes his way downstairs. He opens the front door—and with it, an icy blast. Two sombre-looking policemen are invited inside, just as Mum arrives, carefully adjusting her dressing gown. I remain oblivious, asleep in my cot, as does my brother, Nigel.

"Mrs Adams, we're very sorry to tell you that your mother passed away last night in hospital and as you're not on the phone, we couldn't contact you. We'd like you to come with us to the hospital to identify the body."

"That's ridiculous! There must be some mistake! I saw her only a few days ago and she was fine. She had a bit of a chill, but nothing unusual in this weather. That can't be right!"

"I'm very sorry, but it was flu that turned to pneumonia. And then there were complications in hospital and she couldn't be saved. So if you could get dressed, we'll take you there and an ambulance will bring you back."

Mum can hardly manage the stairs with her head in such a whirl, and Dad doesn't offer to help as he's in shock too. He doesn't bother making a fire so when she returns home an hour later, the house is bitter and bleak and Mum's in despair—and this is just the start.

*

As an adult, my mother told me about this night on several occasions—it was the worst day of her life. After it, she becomes severely depressed for well over a year, and she wasn't able to look after me (at twelve months), or my brother, Nigel, aged five.

As a young child I'm rarely allowed to see her while she's in bed and even when I do, there's no telling what response I'll get. Sometimes it's just silence. Sometimes a brief and difficult cuddle. Usually, I'm glad to leave and go downstairs to play.

When Mum's too depressed to get up, her cousin Emma helps look after us, along with Dad whenever he can take time off from his shops. Emma, like Mum and Dad, is well-meaning, but she's a cool character, an ice-maiden—and maiden she remains, never marrying with no hint of a boyfriend. Like Dad, she believes in strict, old-fashioned ways of child-rearing, especially for boys: no cuddling, leave babies to cry, no unnecessary handling and feed them according to the clock; it's what's 'best' for them, so they don't grow up soft, spoilt and selfish.

Even when Mum's 'better' and I'm a year or two older, our relationship is not great, and if I *do* get a hug or a cuddle, it's often when she's doing something else, like when I sit on her knee as she's stirring the custard, while she's getting dinner ready. But it's never for long before she puts me down again.

So I'm growing up well provided for, but emotionally distant from both parents. In particular, I hate my mother trying to kiss me, even though this is thankfully quite rare. But when she sometimes tries to give me a kiss, normally before bedtime, I hate it and squirm my way out before she manages it, if I can. And then I'm told off for my 'silly' behaviour as I race up the stairs to get out of her way. I expect all this upsets her but I can only feel how I feel, and my feelings run strong.

*

From the very beginning then, we just don't seem to understand or connect with each other. The rest of my extended family are more like Dad—distant, reserved and cool.

Of course, I assume that this is what a *normal family* is like.

2. Cross

"He's a cross!" Know-all Mary shouts aloud as 'Spot' the street dog waddles out to play. "He's a cross between a white dog and a black dog, because he's all white with a big black spot on his back!"

We all laugh, because Mary's quite funny. It's the way she says things. Spot is a really friendly dog who lies on his back to be stroked and tickled, and he takes us for rides on his back, and that's what we decide to do today. So we each get on his back in turn, get hold of his brown leather collar, pat his rear end and shout, "Hi-ho Silver! Away!" Because the Lone Ranger's horse is the only one we all know. So Spot trots off down the street and then returns for the next child, which includes my brother Nigel who, at eight, is a bit big for Spot, but off he goes all the same.

Then it's my turn.

I climb on his back, get hold of his collar, pat his rear and shout, "Hi-yo Silver", just like everyone else and off he trots. But then suddenly, he stops, throwing me forward and I land on my knees in the street. Everyone laughs, then Spot starts to growl and bark at me and chases me down the street, trying to nip my heels. Fortunately, I'm faster than him as I race back to my house, turn left up the side entry and through my back garden gate, which I shut tight behind me. Thankfully, I'm home and Spot is left barking outside, before he gives up and waddles away. I'm frightened, upset and exhausted; I'd never seen Spot like this before—none of us had—so why did he pick on me?

I then look down at my knees. They are grazed, one quite badly with a trickle of bright red blood running down.

"Never mind, Mum will sort it out, she's good at bandaging knees."

I walk down the garden path and go to open the back door, except it won't open. I call out for Mum but there's no reply. It's all eerily silent. I peer through the kitchen window and see the clock—2.15.

And *then* I remember! It's a Thursday afternoon and it's half-day closing for Dad's shops. Mum and Dad have gone out for the afternoon to the countryside—

like they often do in the summer. I wonder what time they will be coming back? Probably about 4 o'clock—that's almost two hours away!

I feel myself getting more and more upset as I check all the back windows, but they are all tightly shut. And I'm not going around the front in case Spot sees me and chases me again. I'm desperate to get in the house, to get some food and drink and to get bandaged up, but it's just not possible. I'm stuck! I hope Nigel comes back to see what's happened to me but there's no sign of him.

So I just sit on the steps and wait…and wait. It's well after 5 o'clock before my parents return. By now, I'm too exhausted with being upset to express the anger I feel inside. In any case, I'd only be told off and sent to my bedroom.

My mother looks at my knees.

"Have you been falling down again? We can't leave you for five minutes without you getting into trouble!"

"But Spot tried to bite me—he chased me all the way home!"

"Spot's a lovely dog. I'm sure he wouldn't bite anyone. Or if he did, then you must have upset him!"

There's no point arguing, because they just won't listen. So I bury my anger and don't tell a soul.

Deep down, I'm upset and hurt. I'm not just cross—I'm livid!

3. Shock and Awe I

"Jamie! Curly! Come here right now! What do you think you're doing?"

It's our headmistress—how unlucky can you get? She gives us a right telling off and tells us to report to her office first thing in the morning, ready for the strap! Ouch! I don't want *that*!

*

At infant school, life is dull, until I team up with Curly who's a bit of an imp and gets himself into more scrapes than me. On the way home, he suggests a game—that we collect some stones and throw them at the passing traffic to see if we can hit a hub-cap or two. The one who hits the most hub-caps is the winner. It sounds great fun and it is for a while, until an old black Austin shudders to a halt and the driver gets out. We start to leg it until we hear old Miss Sanders' familiar voice.

Next morning, we get another stern lecture and, shaking like leaves in a tree, we make our humble apologies. We are shown the strap but it's only applied to the table—*whack*! So we are let off and thankfully, she didn't tell our parents either.

*

The next day, Curly has another idea. I have my doubts, but this time it seems okay. In fact, it sounds brilliant!

"My parents own a sweet shop so let's go and be really nice to them, wash some dishes and then we can have some sweets—for free!" Of course, I'm all for it. So we manage to wash and dry some pots and pans and get our reward from his Mum. She's really nice. And then something seriously weird happens, something I'd never seen before…

Curly's dad pops in from the shop just to say hello, I think. Curly runs up to him and leaps into his arms and they have a cuddle! And then I notice Mr and Mrs cuddling each other—and they kiss! Proper kisses! I'm shocked—*this isn't normal*! Then Curly tells me that it's my turn (in Monopoly) but I don't hear him, because I'm absolutely glued to Mr. and Mrs. And I like what I see, even though it's definitely *not normal*. I'm dead envious too—how nice to live in a family like *that*! I'm in shock and awe of such a lovely, warm and affectionate family and the rest of Monopoly passes me by almost unnoticed.

*

It's a year or so later when I meet Glenda in my new class at junior school. A sweet, pretty girl with a neat, pageboy haircut, white blouse and red tartan skirt with a huge silver safety-pin. She seems to like my 'Sooty' puppet that I've brought to school and suggests we take him for a walk around the school field at lunchtime. I like the idea, especially as it's summer.

Before long, we're walking close to each other as the children's playground chatter subsides into the distance. Glenda's very smiley and suddenly, I want to put my arm around her waist—but do I dare? I take a quick look around to check that no one's watching and then I take the risk; I feel her slender waist in my hand. She gives me another grinning smile and then does the same; I feel her gentle arm around me—bliss! We say nothing for a while and just enjoy the moment, but in time, we relax and start chatting again. It seems the most normal, natural and wonderful thing, to be walking with arms around each other. But we know it's not normal as we've never seen other children do it—especially *a boy and a girl*!

As we approach the school buildings at the end of lunchtime, we let go and pretend nothing has happened. It's our little secret—a secret we re-enact every lunchtime until the term comes to an end and the summer holidays start. On one occasion, a teacher gives us a wink and a grin—he has obviously seen us, but we never hear anything from any of our classmates. They've been too busy playing hopscotch and stuff. Do I tell my parents about Glenda? Not likely!

'Silly, sloppy stuff' they would call it.

That summer, I pass an entrance exam for a Preparatory school for a boys' Grammar the other side of the city and I never see Glenda again—or *any* girls, in fact. The formal character of deference and discipline now reasserts itself at

30

both home and school, as if Curly's family and Glenda never existed. But a glorious interruption to this dour existence is about to come knocking on my door—literally!

4. Shock and Awe II

I've just discovered a new secret world!
But I reckon it's best to keep it that way and not breathe a word to anyone.

*

As Christmas approaches, Nigel and I are told that Mum will be going to work on Saturday mornings, to help out at Dad's shops as trade is good, and that a childminder will be coming to look after us from 10 till 1 o'clock. Her name is Caroline and we must be on our best behaviour, especially for the hour before she arrives, when we'll be on our own. If Caroline reports otherwise, there will be trouble!

*

As Mum and Dad pull out of the drive, our noses are pressed against the front window to watch them go. We wait for a full five minutes to make sure they don't come back. After the five minutes are up, we give a big cheer to celebrate our temporary freedom and waste no time in pushing back all the furniture to the sides of the front room. We put cushions and towels on any sharp corners, and hey presto, we have our own wrestling ring!

We then start to fight and wrestle with each other till shirts and vests come off and faces are beetroot red. Nigel, being older and heavier, usually gets me to 'submit' by kneeling on my arms or giving me a Chinese burn. I get him back sometimes and we never really hurt each other. It's great fun! Ten minutes before our new childminder is due, we put all the furniture back and have a quick wash to hide our red faces. Nigel stays in his bedroom to inspect his butterfly collection and do some of his painting, not wishing to meet her.

As for me, I'm intrigued to find out what our childminder will be like—a change from Mum I hope! I'm still rushing to get dressed properly when she strolls up the drive and rings the doorbell. As I open the door, she laughs at my face, which is still red and sweaty.

"So what have you been up to?"

"We've been having a wrestling match, but please don't tell Mum and Dad!"

"Of course not, so long as there's no blood on the carpet! So let's have a drink and a biscuit, and then you can tell me all about yourself."

I'm warming to her already as she seems really nice. I mean really, really, nice. She looks beautiful as she's tall and slim and pretty with a lovely smile and golden hair up in plaits; red lipstick; a full-length red and white polka dot skirt; a broad, white, shiny, plastic belt around her waist. But most important of all is that smile and her eyes that look straight into mine. I'm feeling a bit overwhelmed as she starts to ask me about myself and my new school. No one has ever asked me stuff like this before so I lap up her attention and am secretly delighted that Nigel is staying up in his bedroom. And suddenly, I recall the warmth, attention and affection that I'd seen at Curly's house, but this time it's all for me!

Auntie Caroline (as I call her) is also great fun and suggests some games to play, such as *Simple Simon Says* and *Playing Dead. Simple Simon Says* gets me very excited, so next she suggests *Playing Dead*, I think to calm me down a bit. First, she lies on the carpet and I've got to see if she moves at all, even a twitch or a blink. Whoever lasts the longest is the winner. After a few minutes, I see her blinking.

"You're not dead!" I shout, and then it's my turn.

So I lie flat on my back and shut my eyes so I don't need to blink. I feel something firm on my chest and reckon it's her foot, with just her stocking on. Then a sort of shadow starts to cover my face—it's her long polka dot skirt— and I realise that if I open my eyes, she wouldn't be able to see me peeking. So that's exactly what I do. I immediately see her foot and, as I continue to gaze upwards, I see her beautiful pinkish legs and the gentle curve of her bum! There's several white strappy things too and other lacy bits. Gosh! It's an awesome sight, and a lot to take in, before I shut my eyes again and allow the game to continue. But my head is in a spin: I've just discovered a new secret world, but I reckon it's best to keep it that way and not breathe a word to anyone.

When Mum and Dad return, I can't wait to tell them how wonderful Auntie Caroline is, how fun she is and how she seems to like me, and I really like her! I thought they would be pleased, but they don't seem to be. I tell them the same after her every visit, but then, after Christmas, suddenly and without warning, another lady comes instead, who's stricter and no fun at all and I never see Auntie Caroline again.

5. Let's Dance

I'm in the dark and feeling lonely. I'm in a boys' dormitory with Nigel at a boarding school in the Warwickshire countryside. We're on a so-called holiday because Mum and Dad have dumped us here while they go off on a proper holiday by themselves. We enjoy holidays with them more than being at home because we do things like play cricket and go on boat trips.

But not this year because we're at a boarding school in the countryside that's run by the County Council. So far it's been pretty awful because everyone else seems to know each other and we don't know anyone. The only good thing is a gaggle of giggly girls, who are a bit older than me. Nigel keeps well away but I am curious, and Melanie, the one with the ponytail, seems very nice; although I'm far too shy to speak to her. So it's cold sausages for breakfast and boring walks each day. No sea and sand, no ice-creams, no boat-trips and definitely no cricket. Just walks—and then Melanie goes and twists her ankle and disappears from sight. We just want to go home and eventually, Friday comes!

But there's a problem, a big problem, one last hurdle to overcome before we get to go home. We've been told there's a 'social' tonight, the last night—can you believe! And we've all got to go, no exceptions. Nigel is refusing as he doesn't want to meet all those children that we've not talked to for the whole week. So he's lying on the bottom bunk with the lights off so that his absence won't be missed. I feel the same too, more or less, but I don't want to be told off for not going, even though I'll hate it. So what to do? If I stay in the dormitory, I'll get lonely as Nigel doesn't talk to me, he just grunts. If I go, I'll be late and then I'll hate it when I get there. In the end, I decide to go—definitely not wanting to be told off.

There's laughter and clapping coming from the hall as I approach, which only makes me feel worse. I keep my head down and manage to shuffle into a back row of chairs without being noticed. Most of the children are seated on the floor watching a clown and when I look up, I can see the gaggle of giggly girls on the far side. Soon, there's a big round of applause for the clown as he takes his bow and my worst fear is realised—it's time for dancing! Feeling impelled to escape and rush back to the dormitory, I edge along the seats and into the corner where, head down, I contemplate my next move. Every second seems like an hour as I plan my escape.

However, as I look up, I get a shock; I'm surrounded by the gaggle of giggly girls and I can see that they are all made-up and looking pretty.

"Come on, Jamie, come and dance with us!"

"I can't dance. Leave me alone! I just want to go home!"

"But we'll teach you, it's easy. Oh come on, don't be a spoilsport!"

At this point, two of them undo the vice-like grip of my hands on the chair, then take me by the hand to the dance. I'm a most reluctant dancer but they persevere and gradually, when I realise that someone is calling out the moves and the music has a good beat, I start to get the hang of it. And as we dance, I find myself dancing with one, then another. All the time I'm trying hard not to actually touch them as I hold on to their dresses between my thumb and forefinger. Then another partner change and with it, a familiar voice and face— it's Melanie! She had gone to hospital to be checked out and was told that it was not a twist but a sprain, to be cured by a few days' rest. Now she's here, with her ponytail and sweet smile, helping me to dance.

"Jamie, just one thing. Let go of my dress and hold me properly, like this," as she wraps my arm around her waist, which pulls me in closer. It's a bit scary but also a delicious feeling, her slender body so close to mine. I want to dance with her some more!

Time has sped by without my realising and my one dance with Melanie is the last of the evening as the music stops and we're all ushered back to our dormitories. As I walk slowly back, I realise how much I enjoyed dancing with the giggly girls and how kind they had been to me. I enthuse about it to Nigel on my return, but he's not in the least bit interested.

"Well, if it was like *that*, I'm even gladder that I didn't go!"

*

Back at home, the emotionally cool, well-ordered and non-tactile regime resumes its familiar dominance, reinforced by Prep school. But the memory lingers of those young giggly girls who had taken care of me and had given me their attention.

I continue to go about my grey half-existence of home, school, homework and a few school friends. I'm well taught at school and well looked after by my parents—at least physically and materially. But life is so very dull…until a bolt from the blue suddenly changes everything!

6. One-Way Ticket

The rusty old turnstile won't budge as I push against it with all the might that a skinny nine-year-old can muster. I panic for a moment, then, with an extra shove, it starts to revolve, creaking and groaning as it moves. At last I'm in! Heralding my arrival is *Neil Sedaka* blaring out of the Tannoy system the rocky sounds of *One Way Ticket*. [3].

I try to work out which way to go. In front of me is a steep grassy bank, so I search for some steps. Above me is an endless sky of blue. As I climb the concrete steps, my excitement mounts, recalling holidays at the coast, expecting a panoramic seascape to appear, but this time it's a football panorama that awaits.

I reach the final step and suddenly, *Wow*! It's a moment that rocks my sheltered world: the vast expanse of the stadium with its concrete terracing, wood and metal grandstands and four towering floodlight pylons. In the middle, uniting the four sides, are the green and brown swathes of the pitch itself, with four corner posts, white perimeter markings and goals at either end. I turn to look behind me and there, rising twice the height of the grassy bank, is the wooden terracing of the *Spion Kop*, for those who want a bird's-eye view of the game.

I have arrived at Highfield Road, the home of Coventry City Football Club, for the very first time.

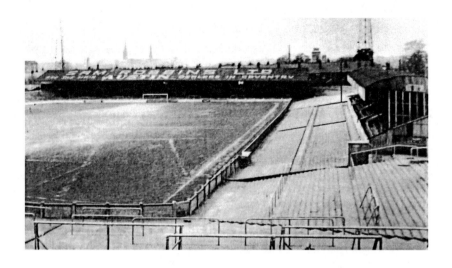

The author's first view of Highfield Road in April 1959

*

Just an hour previously, I had been in my own house, kicking my heels and extremely bored, with nothing at all to do. In sheer desperation, I call out: "Mum, what's a football match like?"

"I've no idea. Better ask your father."

"But he's not here and I want to go—I'm so bored!"

So Mother looks in the local newspaper and discovers there's a match on: *Coventry City reserves v Millwall reserves. Kick-off 3.00 pm.*

As it's a reserve match, there won't be any bustling crowds to trouble me, so she takes me in the car and drops me off near the turnstiles, on the condition that afterwards, I will go straight to my dad's shop, which is only a stone's throw from the ground. Of course, I agree, so here I am!

The players come out and the game starts, but I'm more interested in exploring. I go right to the top of the *Spion Kop*, from where I can see the whole city as well as the stadium. The players are like ants so I skip all the way down the terracing to pitch-side, where the action is right in your face—players shouting, sweating, shirt-tugging and clattering tackles! I walk right around the pitch inside the perimeter wall, until I reach the Main Stand where I'm not allowed in. I watch the game from there for a few minutes before skipping all the way back, pausing to catch glimpses of the action as I go. It's great fun! A wonderful, glorious day! And I'm an immediate football convert!

The game ends 0-0, but I'm not bothered because I love just being there—the freedom to explore, to do exactly what I want for an hour or so—an escape from home with all its rules and restrictions. I love the freedom to feel how I want to feel, and to shout 'bugger' as often as I want when City miss an open goal. Because, at home, if I get excited, my parents will always try to calm me down, or if I'm bored they'll tell me to "buck up". But at football, I can be who I want and feel how I want to feel, so I become 'football crazy' and talk, sleep and dream about nothing else.

*

Dad occasionally goes to night matches so he buys me a season ticket and, for the very first time, we have something in common to talk about—occasionally. Within twelve months of that first match, I'm lucky enough to see Third Division City beat the mighty West Ham 2-1 in the final of a minor Cup competition. Eighteen months later, Jimmy Hill takes over as manager, leading *The Sky Blue Revolution*, which includes a 'giant-killing' F. A. Cup run, promotion to the Second Division and the modernisation of the stadium. Three heady years later and *The Sky Blues* are Second Division champions and promoted to the First Division for the first time in the club's 84-year history. For me, *the Swinging Sixties* are transformed into *The Sky Blue Sixties*. But, even at the height of City's success, there's still something missing from my life (2.1). But what?

7. The First Kiss

Girls don't go to football matches, I'm thinking as I look around at the scattering of old and middle-aged men in the Old Stand at Highfield Road.

It's an evening reserve match under floodlights and the atmosphere is a lot more relaxed than at first team matches. The players are coming out to warm up, when a strange thing happens—a girl about my own age starts making her way along my row and sits herself down two seats away. She's followed by the old guy who sits next to me every game—like me, he's a season-ticket holder. He sits in between us, in his normal seat and introduces me to Chloe, his granddaughter. She has a very modern look with make-up and spiky hair, a leather jacket and a very short skirt. And pretty too, apart from a broken front tooth. I'm intrigued as to why she's here as she looks a bit out of place; though I'm not exactly complaining.

At half-time, her granddad goes off for his regular cuppa so we lean across to chat.

"I've always wanted to know what a football match is like, so Granddad said I should come along with him sometime—and that there's a nice boy who sits next to him—so here I am!"

I'm flummoxed by her directness so I ask her what she thinks of our centre-forward's first-half goal. But she says she didn't notice it, and then asks me if we were winning! Thankfully, her granddad returns to his seat, thus sparing me further awkwardness for the rest of the game. But I'm still intrigued and at the next reserve match, she's back.

This time, she sits in her granddad's seat, right next to me, with Granddad on the other side. While it's nice to have a girl next to me at a football match, I have to lean over her to her granddad to get any sensible discussion about the game. At the end of the match, he offers to give me a lift home as we all live on the same side of the city. He tells us to hop in the backseat and we're soon smiling at each other and then holding hands. Should I try to kiss her? But I can see Granddad looking in his rear mirror, so perhaps not. Before I get out, she invites me to a relative's birthday party, not far from where I live. It seems that I have a girlfriend at last!

It's about a week to the party and I'm thinking about her a lot—and how nice it is to have a girlfriend. Where we shall go? What we shall do? What will Mum and Dad think? But when I arrive at the party, she just says hello to me, then disappears, and I'm left talking with her aunties and uncles and they wonder who I am. A bit later, she reappears, takes me to one side, walks me to the nearest bus-stop and waves me goodbye! I never see her again, but at the matches, I talk strictly about football with her granddad.

Before long, I find myself thinking: *Girls don't go to football matches, and thank goodness for that!*

*

A year later, I'm invited to a teenage party by Danny, my football-mad friend from across the road. We get invited through his sister to equalise girl-boy numbers for her friend's birthday. We arrive a bit late but it seems there are plenty of boys anyway, and couples seem to be pairing up as they head to the kitchen for food. As they emerge with their paper plates full, Danny stops to chat to some of the lads from his football team while I spot a girl who has only just arrived and is looking a bit lost.

Evie is a petite, attractive girl with sharp lines to her navy miniskirt and dark hair in a neat bob. I offer her some of my plate, which is gratefully received, but we've scarcely finished before someone turns the lights off and the music up. As I adjust my eyes, I can see a room full of couples settling into armchairs and corners with large cushions. I also see Danny's silhouette—he's cutting a lonely figure sitting in a chair by himself. For a moment, I wonder if I should offer to share Evie; *forty-five minutes each way and change over at half-time?* But I quickly think better of it and turn my attention to my new party-friend, who seems to be happy enough sitting on my lap within the confines of a large, soft armchair.

It's not long before Evie is wrapping her slender arms around my neck and gently drawing her face closer to mine. I get a whiff of her peachy perfume as her peach-like cheeks brush mine. I'm keen to taste her lipstick as she wiggles her bum in my lap. We hold back for a few seconds until our lips first brush, then caress each other, her mouth widening to anticipate my eager response. You'd think I'd never been kissed by a girl before! Which, of course, I hadn't.

Occasionally, we come up for air and have a quick look around at the various manoeuvres in the dark. Out of the corner of my eye, I notice Danny get up from his chair and leave the room. I feel sorry for him, but what can I do? Then it's back to business with Evie for another hour or so. I wonder about further explorations, perhaps loosening her blouse a bit, but I don't want to risk causing a scene. Of one thing I am sure however, I want to see her again. Surely she'll want to be my girlfriend after such a good evening! But I'll wait for the right moment—at the end of the party.

After the pleasures of two hours of sensuous kissing and cuddling, the lights suddenly go on and parents are back. I nip to the loo then return to get Evie's phone number and address. But she's nowhere to be seen. I look high and low, check on all the bedrooms and search both front and back gardens in case—perish the thought—she's getting off with someone else! I talk to Danny's sister. "Evie? Oh she left straight away, her dad was waiting in the car for her."

I'm devastated and ask everyone who's still there if they know anything about her. But no one does. She's simply vanished into the night without a trace, along with my hopes of a girlfriend, once again. Girls! They can be very nice but you just can't trust them! Anyway, I really enjoyed my first kiss! But it would also be my last kiss, for the time being at least.

8. The Eve of Destruction
Thursday, 25 October 1962

"It's nearly 10 o'clock, Jamie. So off you go to bed, it's school tomorrow."

Hadn't he been listening? Didn't he understand? We might be vaporised by the morning—and school too! I desperately need some reassurance…

"But if I go to bed, will I ever wake up again? Is there going to be a nuclear war?"

"Son, I don't know if we'll wake up in the morning; let's just hope…"

Some reassurance that!

Dad had been born during the First World War, had fought in the Second World War with the RAF, but he inspired no confidence about our surviving the Third, which was about to break out, probably tonight. And this time, it would be thermo-nuclear with nowhere to hide. For the next twenty-four hours, I believed that we were on the eve of destruction.

We'd just finished watching the BBC 9 o'clock news—news we had been glued to for the past week—and it kept getting worse. We'd seen pictures of Soviet Union ships loaded with nuclear missiles approaching Cuba. We'd seen the USA's naval blockade ready to intercept them and we'd heard the Soviets' declaration that any such intervention would be viewed as an act of aggression and would invite retaliation, possibly nuclear. The USA's B-52 bombers were loaded and primed—and within striking range of Moscow—as the world held its breath.

As I wake up the next morning, I'm hugely relieved that I'm not dead. But as we listen to the radio over breakfast, the danger is clearly not over. I sit on the top deck of the No. 6 bus to school, peering out of the window, expecting a missile to burst through the sky at any second, causing a massive conflagration in the city, which would wipe us out in the ensuing firestorm; we'd all seen the newsreels of the horrors of Hiroshima—eyeballs melting and skin ripped away.

The *Cuba Missile Crisis* (as it became known) shakes us all up and for the rest of our schooldays, my friends and I are continually aware of the possibility of nuclear war. A few years later, a housemaster acknowledges this concern at a House assembly by playing a recently released protest song, *The Eve of Destruction* [4], having first distributed the words to the two hundred students present. We're all impressed. It's a powerful yet sombre number by Barry McGuire, which expresses the mood of the Cold War backdrop to our teenage lives in the mid-1960s. Its lyrics about the nuclear button being pressed and the world becoming a graveyard fills us all with dread. At the end of the assembly, we all troop out in funereal silence—it's the only assembly I remember from the whole of my school days.

Then it's back to the joys of Latin, maths and double chemistry.

*

From the time when I started Prep school, I'd begun taking an interest in the news. It was the court case about the publication of *Lady Chatterley's Lover* (1960) that first got me reading my parents' newspaper, *The Daily Express*; although I took great care to conceal my interest in this particular story, suspecting that the content of the banned book was rather rude and would be beyond the pale for my puritanical parents.

Before long, the TV news became more sombre, with newsreel footage of the building of the Berlin Wall, with people jumping from buildings, families being separated and barbed wire going up across the city, with ordinary German citizens being shot if they dared try to cross it. The Cold War had started and I was concerned in case it became a *real* war. Such anxieties increased the following year with the Cuban missile crisis, as the United States and the Soviet Union stared into the abyss of a potential Third World War—only this time it would be nuclear, with Britain being a certain target for Soviet warheads.

There was to be no let-up in Cold War news, as the *Profumo Affair* (1963) revealed that Britain's defence secrets may well have been compromised and leaked to the Russians, and I was worried that they might take advantage of such inside information. However, as I was soon to discover, there was an upside to this particular story as I became absorbed by the sexual antics of Christine

Keeler, Mandy Rice-Davies, John Profumo and Stephen Ward. Again, I made sure that my parents remained ignorant of my interest and I only scoured their newspaper—and the family dictionary—once I was sure they were out of the house. In the dictionary, I looked up the meanings of 'procure', 'call-girl', 'prostitute', 'brothel' and 'osteopath', as the Cold War itself became somewhat overshadowed by this new and exciting world taking place inside my thirteen-year-old head.

*

Six months later, a newsflash interrupts the *Harry Worth Show* to announce that President Kennedy has just been assassinated by a lone gunman, Lee Harvey Oswald, who is believed to be a Russian-Marxist sympathiser. Then, a few days later, in full view of live TV cameras, he too is shot dead. It seems the whole world is going mad, which is later reinforced by the assassinations of Martin Luther King and Robert Kennedy and by the large, and sometimes violent, demonstrations that take place in London and in other capital cities around the world.

Thus, the words of Bob Dylan speak to myself—and even to my parents—as we can all see that *The Times, They Are A-Changin* [5]. This is the world that I and my school friends inhabit and absorb during our teenage years—a frightening and disturbing world that co-exists uneasily with the highs and lows of the Swinging sixties, with its rock, pop, hippies—and Coventry City!

But it's not the only roller-coaster ride that I'm on.

9. Rollercoaster

1966

I'm looking for a girl—a particular sort of girl. A girl who's about my age and who's not stuck, limpet-like, to a boyfriend or to her family's protective cocoon.

*

In the ballroom, the sounds of the sixties are providing the beat, as children, teenagers and families eat, drink and dance. I'm soaking up the atmosphere, but after half an hour, I've realised that the sort of girl I'm looking for are few and far between. I'll give it another fifteen minutes and then I'm out of here and back to the chalet, or the TV room for the football World Cup.

I continue to scan the ballroom, envious of all the boys with a girl in tow. My eye catches a girl with long dark hair and a red plastic miniskirt. She's across the other side of the ballroom and seems to be on her own—and she's looking straight across at me. I hold her gaze for a few seconds before she turns abruptly and pushes through some double doors. For a moment, I'm a rabbit caught in the headlights wondering what to do, before spotting a nearby exit. Outside, I don't want to lose her among all the campers milling around. So I walk quickly, trying hard not to look ridiculous, and soon I spot her bright shiny skirt. I slow my pace down until I catch up with her, then walk alongside for a few seconds before speaking up: "Didn't you like the dance then? I saw you there…"

"I know you did. I saw you too—that's why I left…I'm joking!"

"Do you want to go back? We could have a dance."

"Nah, too many kids. I'd rather walk. Where shall we go?"

We take a left fork and find the camp's perimeter path, but it starts to drizzle so we head back to the chalets. By now, it's eerily quiet and a solitary orange lamp is casting deep shadows among the wooden cabins. When we reach her chalet, the rain has stopped so she takes me by the hand and leads me deep into the narrow alleyway between her chalet and the next, where the lamplight doesn't reach. It's pitch black until our eyes adjust. She has me with my back to the side of the wooden chalet, where she starts to undo my Beatle-style jacket, before sliding her hands inside and around my back.

"My name's Babs by the way. I feel a bit chilly so I'm warming myself up!"

Her face then reaches up to mine and we sip our first tentative kiss, sweet, soft and gentle, with neither of us wanting to pull away. Eventually, I remove my jacket completely and pop it round her bare shoulders. I'm quite warm anyway, sandwiched as I am between the chalet and her pressing body. I feel her leg slip between mine, as her miniskirt rises up and with it, my interest. Having started with lips, we proceed to kiss more deeply while I start to ease her top out of her miniskirt until I can feel and caress the soft, bare flesh of her waist and back. We continue like this without going any further for well over an hour until my mouth aches and my lips feel sore. When we try to part, our bodies feel stuck together, so we re-engage until well after midnight. When we finally manage to tear ourselves apart, we agree to meet up at 7.30 the following evening.

This time, we decide to go for a longer walk, out to the sea-front amongst the circling gulls, lapping waves and a spectacular sunset. We hold on tightly to each other, our progress punctuated by frequent stops to appreciate the sunset, which is just an excuse for further kissing. As we continue our haltering walk, both pace and conversation slow down, but the sensuous bodily experience remains strong, if unspoken.

Back at the chalets, we find our favoured spot from the previous night and carry on from where we had left off, with her legs entangling ever more intimately with mine, as we start to explore the contours of each other's body. After an hour of this, I start to wilt as hadn't slept a wink the previous night and even Danny, my friend and fellow camper, had commented on my sore-looking lips. Now they were starting to sting so I make my excuses and eventually depart the scene after fixing another date.

*

Danny and I had harassed our parents for permission to go on holiday by ourselves as we were now sixteen, and we had chosen a holiday camp on the north Wales coast—where there were sure to be plenty of sports and girls. Danny got into a footy team the day after we arrived but didn't seem so keen on making a play for the girls. He always made excuses like *they're too young* or *they're too old* or *they're out of our league*. His diffidence surprised me but if he was happy chasing footballs, then that gave me the opportunity for chasing some girls. I reckoned I could operate better on my own without a reluctant Danny holding me back.

*

Once again, I hardly sleep at all with my excitement and my aroused state disturbing the night hours. Danny's disappointed that I'd left him for two nights running and that, during the day, my only conversation is about Babs. I'd missed his semi-final match and it hardly registers with me that he'd lost: because I'm just daydreaming about my next date with Babs and finding it impossible to concentrate on anything else. I get myself ready ahead of time, intending to arrive at her chalet a bit early, perhaps getting a sneak of her changing or getting dolled up. I've got a flowery card in which I've written a verse, hoping to impress:

> *Throughout the day it's you I miss,*
> *Evening brings your tender kiss.*
> *At night I think of you and dream,*
> *And hope our love is evergreen.*

It's the first time I've ever written anything like this to a girl and I'm pretty pleased with my efforts. I'm very excited as I approach and as I pass by the end of 'our' little alleyway, I naturally take a peek. But I'm stopped in my tracks as I see another couple there in a tight clinch—and the girl's wearing a bright red miniskirt! I soon realise it's Babs, together with a tall, well-built lad. I quickly move away and seeing a light on in her chalet, I knock gently on the thin wooden door. Eventually, a big surly girl appears. "Yes?"

"I'm meant to be seeing Babs, but—"

"Look! She's with her boyfriend, okay? They fell out a few days ago and she wanted to make him jealous, but now they're back together. So piss off and don't come back!"

I'm shocked, stunned and reeling. Disappointed, dumped and sworn at, all in one go! I'd never been sworn at before, not that I could remember—and certainly never by a girl! I thought girls were sugar and spice and all things nice—not fat, foul-mouthed morons! I'm disconsolate and walk around in circles for ages, trying to understand how anyone could let me down like that. I still have the card in my hand so I open it and re-read the verse, then violently rip it to shreds and throw it in the air to vent my upset and anger. When I eventually return to my own chalet, I'm a bit calmer but still feeling angry, humiliated and empty. Danny tries to cheer me up but without much success. I'm a dead loss with girls; yet the more I get rejected, the more desperately I want a proper girlfriend. It's a vicious circle.

*

Once again, football comes my rescue; it's the World Cup in England and the following day, we play France and win 2-0, which Danny and I watch in one of the camp's TV rooms. That cheers me up and thereafter, I am glued to the competition, with England going on to win the World Cup, as my hunger for a girlfriend temporarily subsides. After the national excitement (and mine) dies down, my home, school and Coventry City routines continue as normal, except that I'm about to start my A levels. Outwardly, things seem much the same as they have been, but I can feel that *I'm* starting to change.

Not so much in my body, but most definitely inside my head.

10. Childhood Attachments: Review

i.   The evacuation of children from British cities started on 1 September
       1939 and continued thereafter in waves. Millions of children's lives were
       affected, as well as the adults who were saying goodbye, and those who
       were to be the recipients of a new and temporary family, whether in UK
       or abroad in Commonwealth countries.

ii.   John Bowlby, an army psychiatrist at the time, was concerned about the
       emotional damage that such separations might have on the children, so
       he conducted some research. His findings, as well as that of others in the
       field, contributed greatly to an understanding of *maternal deprivation*
       and the importance of childhood attachments—findings that have since
       been modified but largely accepted by all those who work in childcare—
       from parents and midwives to teachers and child psychologists. Such
       understanding did not become public knowledge until the sixties, and
       even then there was still much research to be done before a detailed
       picture could be built up of all the factors involved.
       Unfortunately, neither my parents nor my brother nor I would benefit
       from such a revolutionary understanding of the early years of childhood,
       leaving Mum and Dad to continue the authoritarian child-rearing
       traditions that had been modelled by their own parents.

iii.   Nigel, born four years earlier than myself, was the first to feel the effects
       of our parents' harsh regime of a highly regulated, unaffectionate and
       non-tactile upbringing. Gender would have played its part, as emotional
       distance and lack of affection was deemed necessary to make a boy
       become a man. Boys were routinely left to cry, rarely picked up or
       cuddled and never told they were loved, even if they were. It was
       presumed that any other course would lead to spoilt, selfish and weak
       young men. Nigel became emotionally detached from both parents—

what attachment theory later recognised as *insecure avoidant attachment,* which is brought about by serious emotional neglect. Of course, our parents thought they were doing the right thing, for that is how they had been brought up themselves. There was plenty of respect for authority but an absence of warmth and affection within both our nuclear and extended family networks.

iv. With a second child, our parents may have eased up a bit with their harsh regime, but Mum's traumatic loss and subsequent depression (1.1) would not have allowed for such a possibility. At just twelve months, I was at the age when young children start to bond with and form emotional attachments to their primary carers, so Mum's severe and lengthy depression would have had a number of troubling effects. Being lost in her own grief, functioning at all with Nigel and myself (a needy one-year-old) would have been difficult for her. For the next two years, she was not able to be reliable, affectionate or sensitive to our needs, as any sensitivity would have been for her own needs as she tried to cope with her continuing grief. There was no opportunity for either of us to become securely attached to either Mum or Dad, for that requires reliability, emotional warmth, physical affection and sensitivity.

v. With Mum upstairs in bed for much of the time, Dad needed to look after us more than he had been expecting. From his point of view, strict child-rearing, with minimum contact and affection and maximum adherence to rules was just what the situation required. But most weekdays, he was out at work so they asked Mum's cousin Emma if she could help, which she did. But she too was a cool and distant character with traditional ideas of child-rearing similar to Dad's, so the authoritarian nature of our upbringing was reinforced, resulting in my childhood being characterised by inner loneliness, anxiety and confusion.

vi. As Bowlby's research suggested, those crucial first years laid down an *internal working model* in a child's brain, about how loveable they were and what treatment they could anticipate from adults in the future. According to the typology of Mary Ainsworth (Bowlby's collaborator), I became *anxious-ambivalently attached,* as I swung between my desperate need for love and affection and my inner rage when these needs were not met. More detailed research has revealed that anxious-ambivalent attachment is the result of inconsistent parenting—typical of which would be a new mother suffering from clinical depression, who can only nurture her child in fits and bursts and often from a sense of guilt as she tries (in vain) to make up for lost time. In this manner, mother and child become emotionally out of tune with each other.

vii. Given this background, it's hardly surprising that I was shocked when, at Curly's house, I witnessed the open display of affection between his parents and Curly, the likes of which I had never seen before. Shocked, but also deeply envious, as it was such affection that I longed for but hardly ever received. Neither is it surprising that when I was befriended by Glenda at junior school (1.3), I was delighted to hold and be held by another human being, especially a pretty girl.

viii. When 'Auntie Caroline' arrived at our house as a childminder (1.4), I immediately sensed that her sort of care was what I had been missing for all of my young life. The questions she asked, the eye contact and smiles she made and the fun and hugs she gave me were all in stark contrast to the emotionally withheld, non-tactile and humourless atmosphere of our parental home. In particular, it was her sensitivity to my needs that drew me to her so that by the end of her first visit, I had fallen in love with the best Mum I never had. This concurs with the research findings of Mary Ainsworth and others that the single main predictor of secure attachment is the *sensitive responsiveness* of the parents/carers towards the child, or the similar concept of interactional synchrony whereby parents and baby learn to 'turn-take' with their responses in harmony with each other: they are making tunes together or 'singing from the same hymn-sheet'—and the child feels understood.

ix. Similar themes can be found in the story of the 'social' that I attended while on an enforced holiday away from my parents (1.5). It was another example of a positive encounter with girls who offered me a rare tactile experience by means of a dance. In fact, the most fondly remembered moments of my early childhood seem to revolve around these three events: Glenda, Auntie Caroline and the dance girls. They all involve young girls or women and all take place away from the presence of my parents. However, these three experiences also had a downside, in that they ended as quickly as they started, and without any warning. In attachment terms, although these girls were emotionally warm, tactile and responsive, they were not *reliable* due to the surrounding circumstances beyond their control. Together with my mother's unreliability, they may have reinforced an internal working model with the following script: *Females, whether family or friends, young or old, are simply not reliable. To depend on them for one's emotional well-being is to take a great risk.*

So perhaps it's not surprising then that my first positive and reliable attachment was to be something entirely different…

x.   Without doubt, the most memorable event of my first decade was my joyous discovery of football in general, and of Coventry City F. C. in particular, when I was nine years old (1.6). My new passion, indeed my first real passion, made everything that had gone before pale into insignificance. With the discovery of Coventry City at Highfield Road, I suddenly felt that I belonged, with a cause and a purpose. I also delighted in the freedom from parental control that this new-found passion offered, for although my father was an occasional City supporter himself, we rarely attended matches together. Following the City gave me the emotional freedom to express my feelings how *I* wanted, without being told to 'buck up' or 'calm down' by my regulatory parents.

Watching Coventry City did not offer an immediate tactile experience (except when they scored) and few girls were to be seen at matches. But these limitations were far outweighed by all the benefits, so I soon became a season-ticket holder and remained so for most of my teenage years, including following the team to away matches from time to time, usually by myself.

xi.   In psychological terms, I had discovered a positive substitute attachment that superseded the very poor quality attachment that I had with my parents. Yet the very passion with which I followed *The Sky Blues* (as they became known) was in fact generated by my anxious-ambivalent

54

attachment: ambivalence literally meaning strong (valiant) in two (*ambi*) directions. The negative strength was my inward (and occasionally outward) resistance [6] to my parents, with the positive strength being, firstly, towards Auntie Caroline and then, overwhelmingly, to Coventry City. It was a pattern that would repeat itself throughout my teenage and adult life. It would be forever a driven, passionate life, with my early childhood crises being but a microcosm of my life ahead.

xii.   It might be thought somewhat strange that a football club could act as a surrogate or substitute attachment for a parental figure. However, Bowlby and other attachment researchers suggest that institutions such as nation, sovereign, church, hospitals, religion, work and nature [7] can all function in attachment-related ways for some individuals. They have become *institutional attachments* —especially for those who are insecurely attached to their primary caregivers.

xiii.   The ways by which institutions may function as substitute attachments are through their *reliability and availability* and the subjective feelings of security that this engenders. Such institutions may be relatively consistent in the way they deal with individuals, i.e., according to rules rather than by personal predilections. Being of a corporate nature, they may also give rise to a sense of belonging and even personal identity. In these ways, a football club can fulfil some important aspects of an attachment figure for its supporters.

xiv.   However, there is an important limitation with an institution acting as an attachment figure: an institution is not a person. Therefore, although an individual may be attached to the institution, the institution will not be bonded to that individual in the personal way that most (but not all) parents become bonded to their children. Accordingly, the institution may be neither *sensitive nor responsive* to the individual's specific needs, and this could explain why an institution may be ultimately rejected by an individual as a suitable surrogate attachment figure.

Summary:

My early childhood was significantly affected by three main crises:

1. My mother's traumatic experience concerning her own mother's death, which led to her long-term depression and inability to form secure emotional bonds with either Nigel or myself.
2. My development of an insecure-ambivalent attachment to both my parents, which is in part responsible for the emergence within me of other passionate attachments [8].
3. My discovery of Coventry City, which provided me with an alternative, substitute, institutional attachment—and an all-consuming passion for most of my teenage life.

*

To support positive mental health:

1. Children need to be brought up by parents or carers who are reliable, loving, sensitive and affectionate. This will nurture children into having a secure sense of self, which will help mitigate any damage caused by any Adverse Childhood Experiences (ACES) such as poverty, abuse, bullying, divorce or other detrimental events or circumstances.
2. Parents need to guard against physical and emotional neglect, distance or inconsistency. If they don't feel 'in tune' or emotionally connected to their infant offspring, then they should seek help themselves in order to understand the underlying issues they may have unwittingly brought to parenthood.
3. For children and adolescents suffering from an emotional disconnect with their parents and wider family, institutional attachments may provide a positive alternative that will help boost self-esteem, aid sociability and help provide a sense of positive identity. There are literally thousands of such social groups in most advanced societies—including sports and fitness clubs, charitable and environmental organisations and a plethora of educational and community groups.
4. However, as is the case with some parents, some institutions may provide a negative (rather than positive) influence on young lives—as

with street and drug gangs and extremist political, religious and racist movements. By attaching to such groups, an individual's mental health is likely to deteriorate in the long run, despite any initial boost it may provide, through belonging to a welcoming group.

Chapter 2 ~ Religious Crises
1964–86

1. A Still Small Voice
Saturday, 25 April 1964

The ball hits the back of the net for the only goal of the game!

My *Sky Blue* hero and the darling of the terraces, George Hudson, has just helped City win the Third Division Championship for the first time in almost three decades—in front of 36,000 ecstatic fans who roar their approval and delight. As the final whistle sounds, the terrace crowds surge onto the pitch and manager Jimmy Hill leads a raucous rendering of the *Sky Blue Song* [9]:

> *Let's all sing together, play up Sky Blues!*
> *While we sing together, we shall never lose…*

The crowd stays on the pitch and the stands remain full, long after the game has ended. I'm stuck in my season-ticket seat, but I'd rather be on the pitch with the players and where the champagne is flowing. I'm looking in from the outside, but I want to be on the inside. I want to be more involved, more part of the action than just being a happy spectator. I'm overwhelmed by a feeling of wanting to be close, though close to who or what I'm not so sure. Right in the midst of the collective euphoria, I'm suddenly feeling empty and alone.

Perhaps someone is trying to tell me something, but with the ongoing excitement of the *Sky Blue Revolution* and the swinging sixties, it's easy to ignore—for the time being.

*

Later that summer, on the way home from buying *A Hard Day's Night* LP [9a], I hear that inner voice again. It's another footballing drama but of a very different kind. As I pop into a newsagent's for a paper, I see on a front page in bold type: ***John White killed by lightning.***

61

John White was a leading figure of Tottenham Hotspur's trophy-winning team of 1961-3 and a Scottish International—whom I greatly admired after watching Tottenham's two televised F. A. Cup Final victories from those years. He was only a slip of a lad, but a wonderful, classy, inside forward, nicknamed 'the Ghost', for he was elusive and would drift past opposition players as if he wasn't there. Now suddenly, he *really* wasn't there. Gone, after a lightning bolt had killed him while he was playing a summer's round of golf in north London. Such a terrible loss, as that same pang of emptiness and loneliness surges through me once more.

I soon recover my equilibrium and forget about the voice that has caught me off-guard, for the second time in a few months. After all, I've *A Hard Day's Night* to play and enjoy as both my exciting pop world and City's *Sky Blue Revolution* continue their ascendancy.

But the voice from my inner wilderness refuses to remain silent for long. And when I hear it for a third time, it's not just a small voice I hear but a whole conversation—a conversation that leads to a conversion, which will turn my world upside down and change my life forever.

2. The Hollow Men
1965

The book lands with a thud on my desk: *Selected Poems. T. S. Eliot.*

Oh no, not poems! I think to myself. *All clouds and daffodils.* None of us had been taught by Mr Nicholls before, with his crimped white hair and crumpled black gown. The poems are our first set text in A-level English literature and he tells us to have a quick read through of the first one. So it's heads down and eyes fixed for *The Love Song of J. Alfred Prufrock*:

Let us go, through certain half-deserted streets,
The muttering retreats
Of one-night cheap hotels. [10]

And not a daffodil in sight! I'm impressed—it's a good start.

The following week, we move on to *The Waste Land*—almost impossible to understand, yet full of evocative and depressing imagery:

I think we are in rats' alley
Where the dead men lost their bones. [11]

Nickers (as we call him) informs us that it's about decadent western society after the First World War. It seems almost contemporary to me and reminds me of current protest songs such as *The Eve of Destruction* and Dylan's *Times They Are A-Changin* [12]. I ask Nickers whether Eliot's poems and Bob Dylan's songs have stylistic similarities. He gives me an ice-cold stare, says nothing and then, after an audible sigh, moves on. Clearly, he has never heard of Bob Dylan [13].

Next up is *The Hollow Men*, and suddenly the poetry becomes personal for me:

We are the hollow men
We are the stuffed men
Leaning together
Headpiece filled with straw. Alas! [14]

It's no longer about decadent western society—but about decent, yet empty, me. It's good that someone else experiences these hollow, isolating feelings I have inside and has put it in print for all to see. I feel consoled and wonder what's coming next.

After half-term, the lessons move on to what Nickers calls 'the more positive and hopeful' aspects of Eliot's poetry. These poems include *Ash-Wednesday*, *The Journey of the Magi* and *The Choruses from 'The Rock'*, all of which have an unmistakably religious tone. It's the last poem that gets my serious attention as it seems rooted in my experience of everyday life:

Nor does the family even move about together,
But every son would have his motor cycle,
And daughters ride away on casual pillions. [15]

Eliot, himself a convert to Anglican Christianity, offers an antidote to this social disintegration:

You, have you built well, have you forgotten the cornerstone?
Talking of right relations of men, but not of right relations of men to GOD.
[16]

He seems to be suggesting that a renewal of a spiritual Christianity would heal:

a world confused and dark and disturbed by portents of fear [17].

And one place that such spirituality can be located is in the church:

We thank Thee for the lights that we have kindled,
The light of altar and of sanctuary;
Small lights of those who meditate at midnight...

...O Light Invisible, we glorify Thee! [18]

*

I'm intrigued and fascinated by Eliot's evocative religious imagery, as well as by the mysterious *Stranger* in the Rock Choruses, who I take to be an enigmatic Christ-figure. Eliot's world seems to offer a breadth and depth of meaning that is missing from my world of football, Coventry City and pop. So one Sunday evening, I set forth on an Eliot-inspired pilgrimage to the 'altar and sanctuary' of my local parish church. It is here that I become, like Eliot before me, an enthusiastic convert to Christianity as I discover a new teenage identity...and destiny.

3. God's Evangelist
1967

"Don't mention the Bibles! Look who's coming on board!"

It was true—at the first train station after crossing the border into East Berlin, several East German guards climb on board and look around. We all look down at our feet, our hearts racing, for our clothes are stuffed with German New Testaments that we're smuggling across the border to an East German evangelical church on the outskirts of the divided city. It's the height of the Cold War, and we had visited the Berlin Wall earlier that day, with its sombre charred crosses marking the places where would-be escapees had been shot dead.

Mercifully, without being searched, we finally reach the appointed *Evangelische Kirche*. Darkness surrounds us. But when the church doors are flung open, our youth group of twenty with our two Anglican ministers, are greeted with open arms, tears and a fulsome hot meal. They had recently had all their Bibles confiscated by the communist authorities and were delighted when we all pulled out about five New Testaments each. After food, fellowship and prayers in both languages, we set off back to the bright lights of West Berlin, now relieved of our contraband as well as our anxiety as we cross back from east to west. Of all the bright lights, none shines more brightly for me than the azure blue interior of the Kaiser Wilhelm Memorial Church with its luminous, large, gold crucifix above the candle-lit altar—and I wish that Celia, my new girlfriend from my local Baptist church [3.1], was with me to share these evangelistic and spiritual experiences.

*

However, this is not the only mission I am engaged in, for I now belong to three different Christian youth groups in Coventry—not being one to do things by halves. My second group has an ongoing mission to the 'rocker' cafés along a three-mile stretch of one of the city's arterial roads. Before the Berlin trip, we went out to these cafés two nights a week, dressed in all black, to talk to the rockers about Jesus and the difference He can make to one's life. Although we were initially fearful of their fierce reputation, they seemed to respect us and our mission. We even got front-page coverage in the *Coventry Standard*.

So we invite the rockers back to 'our place' on Sunday nights, at a local church hall. After the elderly congregation has scuttled away, up roar twenty or thirty Harley Davidsons and park in the church carpark. In full leathers, the rockers avail themselves of the armchairs, food, non-alcoholic drinks and toilets—and listen to what we have to say before coming back with their questions and arguments. Occasionally, Noel strikes up with his guitar—he's an expert guitarist and a recent convert—and the hall vibrates to *Amazing Grace* and other rousing evangelical songs. A couple of rockers become 'born again' Christians and join our group. The vast majority do not, but we have witnessed for Christ and we can do no more than that. And off roar the Harleys into the night.

*

My third group is based loosely around the Anglican Church to which I had first set forth on my Eliot-inspired pilgrimage. I had recently attended a Billy Graham rally at Earls Court and I had 'gone forward' at the altar-call at the end. I told my local vicar about this and although not an evangelical himself, he declared that "every parish needs its own Billy Graham."

I had already proved myself a confident speaker at the local Baptist youth group, so I now see myself as 'God's Evangelist' for my own parish. Therefore, with the vicar's blessing and with help from my recently converted friends, I set about organising an evangelical rally in the parish church. I have a specially-made platform for my pulpit, and Noel, a drummer friend of his, plus four teenage girls, including Celia, together form an inspirational and harmonic music group. All I lack is Billy Graham's southern American drawl, but I can, and do, preach the same gospel of 'Christ Crucified' [19]. The Saturday night event is widely advertised, the church is packed and a number of people are converted to Christ, as I am later informed. The following week, 'high on Jesus' and believing 'rock and pop' to be the music of the devil, I give the whole of my extensive pop collection to charity, preferring to sing along to *The Billy Graham London Crusade Choir* [20]. It's the only music I need.

*

I now see my destiny as a full-time evangelist. My vicar tells me to slow down and go to university first—but why waste three years studying when I can be saving souls *now*? I consult with other vicars and ministers, but they all say the same—go to university or at least to a Bible College first. So I'm caught in a real dilemma, for I want to preach and save souls, not study.

However, *"Everything works together for good, for those who love God"* [21], and so, on the boat-crossing back from the Berlin trip, I receive some good news from one of the Anglican ministers with us. He tells me about a college at the University of Durham that has an evangelical tradition, with tuition in theology, which helps prepare students for an evangelical Anglican ministry! I see this as a 'divine calling' for God's evangelist! So I apply for a place and am accepted upon interview.

I'm on my way to St John's College, Durham; praise the Lord!

4. Battle for the Mind I
1968–9

Two police helicopters disturb the early morning calm over Durham city as I leave my digs for the ten-minute walk to breakfast at St John's. One seems to be hovering over the prison and the other across the river, above the Cathedral area close to St John's. I hear the wailing of police sirens as they race through the city's narrow streets and I wonder what the commotion is about. I quicken my walk as I enter South Bailey where I am stopped by a police cordon. They allow me through, but there are police on the steps of St John's, as well as in the dining hall itself. Through the large bay windows I see more police with tracker dogs combing the quad and college lawns. Breakfast has not even started; what on earth is going on?

Suddenly, a spoon is banged loudly at the top table and the room falls silent as the chief inspector strides in and reads out a prepared statement:

"Ladies and gentlemen, last night several dangerous prisoners escaped from the maximum security block, E-wing, at Durham prison. Two have already been recaptured but one remains at large. We have reason to believe that, late last night, his escape route took him through these college gardens and outbuildings. He may still be in the vicinity, lying low.

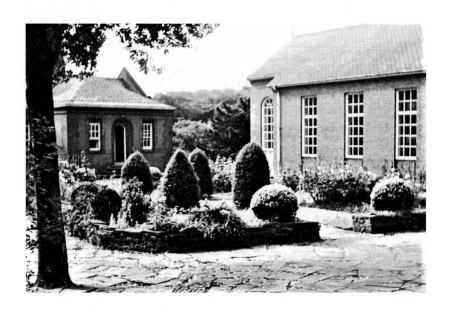

St. John's College, Durham. The quad, as it was in 1969.

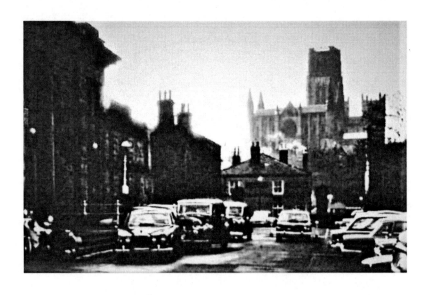

The forecourt of HM Prison, Durham,
the scene of McVicar's escape October 1968.

"Therefore, I strongly suggest that you go about your business today in groups of two or more, and not by yourself as this man is extremely dangerous. If you see or hear anything suspicious, do *not* approach him but call us on 999.

His name is John Roger McVicar, and posters with his photograph are going up around the city as I speak. A police cordon is also in place on all roads leading out of the city. Please do not go far from this college today, as we will need to interview every one of you, without exception, before the day is out.

Thank you for your cooperation." [22]

There is a collective intake of breath after the chief inspector leaves. The interviews start straight away. For the rest of the week, we all sleep uneasily in our beds until we learn that the manhunt has switched to London. We remain bemused; how anyone could escape from the infamous 'E-wing' at Durham Prison, the front carpark of which I walk through twice a week en route to lectures. Weeks later, we hear that McVicar still remains at large; although, it's thought, no longer in Durham. We all breathe a collective sigh of relief and college life resumes as normal—but not for me.

*

I'm now in my second term at John's and I've already undertaken several local preaching engagements at outlying Anglican and Methodist churches. On the college notice-board, I'm struck by a poster about an Open Lecture on a Friday night, entitled 'Battle for the Mind'. It has been arranged by the Anthropological Society, whose president was my friendly student mentor when I first arrived at St John's. He's also a keen evangelical Christian. The lecture is by William Sargant, a leading London psychiatrist, and it takes place in the green-roofed Appleby lecture theatre on the science campus. It looks like an interesting topic and the lecture hall is packed.

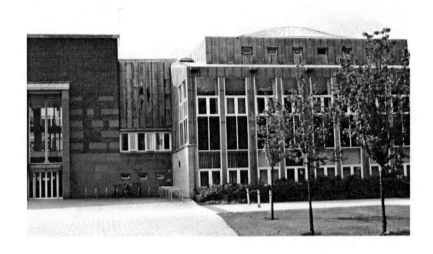

The Appleby lecture, Durham—and 'The Battle for the Mind' lecture, 1969.

Dr Sargant illustrates his talk by film-clips of initiation rituals of African and Indonesian tribes, at which individuals are induced into a state of ecstasy prior to their conversion into the tribe's religion. He emphasises the power of group suggestion, the rhythmic drumming and chanting and the induced emotional excitement that appears to promote the ecstatic state, trance and ensuing conversion. Although his focus is on non-western tribes, he makes passing reference to snake-handling sects in America, the revivalist mass conversions of John Wesley (with which I am well acquainted) and the modern conversion techniques of Billy Graham.

I suddenly find myself with conflicting thoughts. I was not converted at the Billy Graham rally itself, but over a year beforehand through the religious poems of T. S. Eliot. More of an intellectual than an emotional conversion. Nevertheless, my emotions had been engaged and the thought had now been implanted in my brain that religious experiences can easily be explained as psychological processes. So, if my religious experience (upon which I had built my faith) has a purely psychological cause, then what does this mean for the 'indwelling Holy Spirit', for 'Jesus in my heart' and indeed, the very existence of God Himself? As the lecture finishes and chattering students leave the theatre for the pub, I remain immobile in my seat, drowning in doubt.

*

I return to my digs deeply disturbed and depressed, my mind racing. I long for sleep and that I will wake up the morning with my world back to normal—hoping it's all a bad dream. But I awake in the same depressed state, with the same persistent thoughts—that my conversion had been purely psychological and that God does not exist. I am traumatised by such thoughts and my performance for St John's College football team that afternoon is woeful as my eyes are rarely on the ball and I'm forever looking skywards into a now godless universe.

To compound my problem, all my friends, both at home and college, are evangelical Christians for whom radical doubt is an unmentionable sin. So I have no one to talk to about my mental pain and acute distress. I even consider the possibility that *all* our thoughts and behaviours are psychologically or culturally determined, and that free will is itself an illusion along with God [23]. Therefore, humans are just very complex animals, on a lonely planet, in a meaningless universe.

My depression deepens as I consider the ramifications of my sudden unbelief. What should I do about my degree course in theology? What about my vocation to evangelistic preaching and Anglican ministry? My Christian friendships? And Celia, my lovely Christian girlfriend back home? The obvious and honest answers are all too bleak to contemplate.

I then recall a familiar biblical text, which triggers a single positive thought:

Beloved, do not be surprised at the fiery ordeal which comes upon you to test you, as though something strange were happening to you. But rejoice in...Christ's sufferings [24].

*

I start to reframe my situation as a test from God that will make me a stronger Christian and which will, in due time, pass by. At least it's a possibility and worth hanging on to. With this thought in mind, I make four practical resolutions:

1. To advise St John's that I am no longer available for preaching assignments, for the time being.

73

2. To not tell anyone of my doubts but to continue as normal with college and church life.

3. To avoid giving any hint of my problems to Celia, either through my letters or when with her at home. She is a lovely girl with an unquestioning faith. The last thing I want to do is to undermine her faith as well—for I now need her love and affection more than ever.

4. To speak to the president of the Anthropological Society, to see if the lecture has had any effect upon *his* evangelical faith—and how, if possible, he might be able to help me.

He is the only person that I will confide in. As for everyone else, I will hide my doubts and work hard on my acting skills. Perhaps having to pretend is part of the test. Perhaps having these doubts is my 'calling' to share in 'Christ's sufferings' in the modern age.

Though I hardly feel like 'rejoicing', more like jumping off a cliff.

5. Battle for the Mind II
1969–71

The sky is blue and the air is fresh with pine as the congregation spills out of the large wooden chalet near Villars, a township a thousand feet above Lake Geneva in the Swiss Alps. As I greet the rugged-looking pastor with his thinning hair and trimmed goatee beard, I take his hands into mine and look directly into his eyes: "Thank you for restoring my faith, and for saving my life."

"Thanks for telling me. I'm glad we could help," he replies with a warm American accent and smile.

This pastor is no ordinary pastor, but Dr Francis Schaeffer, Christian philosopher, author of many books and founder of *L'Abri* [the shelter], an evangelical Christian community for enquiring minds from across the world, religious, non-religious and those still searching for life's meaning [25].

I have just graduated from St John's, Durham, and I'm on a pilgrimage to L'Abri to mark my return to faith more than two years after it was shattered by William Sargant's lecture. It had been a long, arduous and rocky road.

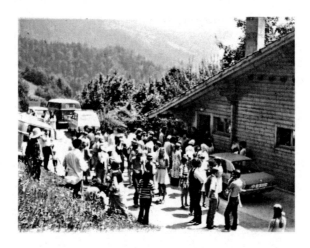

Outside the chapel of L'Abri, a Christian community in Switzerland.

*

As for my four resolutions, I managed to keep them all, including the level of deception necessary to maintain my place within the Christian fellowship at St John's and in the Christian Union, while I beavered away at trying to recover a few fragments of a lost faith.

The outcome of my conversation with the president of the Anthropological Society was that he advised me to focus on my New Testament studies and the reality of the historical Jesus: "For if that is real, then no amount of psychology can undo it." It seemed good advice, so I started to study the Bible for an hour each day in addition to my lectures, tutorials and essay-writing. So I didn't go out very much—hardly at all in fact, until the third term of my final year.

In the early days of my attempts at faith-restoration, I started to develop my faith 'by proxy'. I was aware that many clever and able people, including scientists and psychiatrists, were able to both believe in their professional research and remain Bible-believing, evangelical Christians. Therefore, I reasoned, if *they* can believe, then surely I can too. I had faith in their faith, as it were. A small step in the right direction, it seemed.

Some fellow John's students were concerned about my head being buried in books all the time, so they sought to introduce me to their more charismatic faith, with 'speaking in tongues' and being 'baptised in the Holy Spirit'. However, after William Sargant's lecture, I had no time at all for a faith based on so-called 'spiritual experiences', knowing that there were probably psychological reasons that could explain them. I needed something far more solid and reliable to put my trust in. A faith without any loopholes—where doubt could never enter.

To this end, I was attracted to another tradition within the college, which was followed by the more scholarly and serious students. This was the 'Reformed tradition', which consisted of three key elements: 1. A belief in Biblical inerrancy—that there are no errors of fact in the Bible. 2. A belief in the Bible-based teachings of John Calvin, the supreme Protestant Reformer. 3. The necessity of understanding 'systematic theology' to ensure that one held a complete, unified and logical system of belief—unlike those 'woolly' charismatics! So I proceeded with my studies along these lines and started to develop an authentic faith of my own, which rested on more solid ground.

I then have a lucky break. Or perhaps it's God's hand at work!

It's a typical Saturday evening at the Christian Union, the high spot of which is an hour's talk by a leading evangelical minister. The lecture hall is packed with two hundred students and after it's over, we all mill around in the foyer, as people sort out who's holding coffee parties and in which colleges.

For once, I'm not interested in any coffee parties, despite the attractive young ladies who will be attending. I'm looking at the bookstall, and at one book in particular: *Escape from Reason* by Francis A. Schaeffer [26].

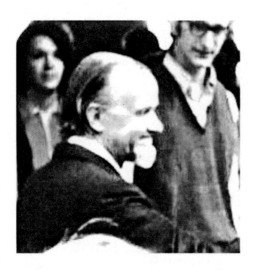

Francis Schaeffer—Christian Philosopher

It's the first Christian book I've come across with the word 'reason' in the title. It's a slim volume that I flick quickly through before buying it. It's packed with diagrams and new ideas, and names like Plato, Sartre, Camus and the Beatles jump off its pages. It's exciting, intellectual and hip—like nothing I've seen before. I race back to St John's with my new treasure and rapidly consume *Escape from Reason* as though I'd not eaten for months. Then a thorough re-read the following morning, instead of college chapel. The book's basic argument is that mankind can't reason its way to God, as most Medieval theologians, such as Thomas Aquinas, tried to do. But if we pre-suppose that God exists, then the world and life's meaning start to make more sense. These hundred or so pages also introduce me to philosophy, society, art and culture, which Schaeffer uses to illustrate his various themes. There is also an added bonus—for it becomes clear that he too is from the Reformed tradition within evangelical Christianity—which confirms the pathway I was already taking.

A few months later and Schaeffer's next book is released: *The God Who Is There* [27], a weightier tome that explicates more fully his previous book. Then *Death in the City* [28]—more sermonic in style. Soon after, an associate of Schaeffer's publishes *Modern Art and the Death of a Culture* [29], a Christian philosophy of art history. It's an exciting intellectual world that I've entered, as Schaeffer's ideas become a central topic of conversation both in college and at Christian Union coffee parties.

*

Towards the end of my time at Durham, a second-year John's student and a young lady from St Mary's take me out punting on the River Wear—the river that surrounds the cathedral and various colleges. Afterwards, we go to the Student's Union for a drink and a bar-snack. As I sup my half of lager and bite into my cheese roll, I'm struggling to hold back the tears. My friends notice and I explain: "You know, this is the first time I've ever been to the Union bar in all my time at Durham."

"It's the first time I've eaten out of college. At last I'm doing something normal, having spent so much time in books. It's like I've been in prison—an intellectual prison of my own making—but I've not really *lived*."

"But Jamie, you've won your battle for the mind, you've overcome your doubts, and no battle is ever easy. But now you're free, so go and enjoy your pilgrimage to L'Abri."

They are very kind and caring friends—and it's an exceptionally tasty cheese roll.

Upon my arrival in Switzerland and L'Abri, I have a strong sense—almost a premonition—that this pilgrimage will mark for me, the end of doubt and that it will be upwards and onwards from now on…

However, before long I come to realise that this is **not** the end.
It is not even the beginning of the end.
It is perhaps, the end of the beginning.
For, unbeknown to me, a far greater conflict lies ahead.

6. Go to Hell

Six years later: 1977–80

It's dark and drizzling as three lanes of traffic speed out of Leicester in the rush hour. As it's an unfamiliar city to me, I'm just going with the flow when suddenly everything goes black and I can't breathe. My heart is racing, I'm out of control and overwhelmed by terror as I prepare for an almighty pile-up. I hit the brakes hard and the car spins around, but amazingly, no one hits me. Just a lot of blaring horns and flashing lights. Just as suddenly, my sight returns but I've got to get across the traffic and stop, which somehow I manage to do. I've had a lucky escape.

I turn off the engine and heave a sigh of relief. I'm soaked in sweat and still shaking. I wait twenty minutes till the traffic, and my panic, subsides before pulling gently away. I realise that I've just had a panic attack, something that I've never experienced before. But why?

*

It's been six years since I left St John's. In that time, I've gained a Cambridge MA, been ordained into the Church of England and have served in a Lincolnshire parish. But parish life didn't suit me. So I'm currently at a Teacher Training College near Lincoln, where I met Sophie, my new girlfriend. But I've other career options as well, and I went to Leicester for an interview for the post of travelling secretary for the Inter-Varsity Fellowship (IVF)—the main evangelical student organisation in the country that supports university and college Christian Unions.

As I continue my journey home, I soon realise the reason for my panic attack; namely that my interview was too successful! I have been invited for a second meeting with a view to being offered a post. I should be pleased, but I'm not, and it's all to do with 'Biblical Inerrancy'—that the Bible contains no errors of fact.

My would-be employers are very hot on this and I knew I would be questioned in detail, which I was. But recently, I've started to 'wobble' about this belief and I felt that my honest answers in the interview were somewhat vague and lacking in conviction.

So I was surprised to be told how well I had performed and that a job was in the offing.

Superficially, I was pleased that I'd done so well. But I felt that I had pulled the wool over their eyes—and over mine too. My unconscious mind, however, was not so easily fooled and protested by means of a panic attack. I now had to face the truth—that I didn't really want the job—at least, not with 'Biblical Inerrancy' tied to it, like an albatross around one's neck. Hand on heart, I just couldn't believe it anymore, so the next day I replied to the IVF, politely turning down the invitation to a further meeting.

A few months later, I am offered a post as chaplain and RE teacher at an independent school near Grantham, and I gladly accept. Here, the chaplaincy has a broad church tradition and my first sermon is about the recent death of Elvis Presley. I've had a lucky escape—two, in fact.

*

It's 1979 and New Year's Eve. Sophie and I are attending an evening service with some friends at their Methodist chapel. Mrs Thatcher, born and brought up in Grantham, has been Prime Minister for some six months, so when she gets a mention in the sermon, my ears prick up:

"We don't know what the New Year will hold for our own Margaret Thatcher, but I tell you this, *your* future will be in eternal hellfire and damnation unless you repent of your sins and accept Jesus Christ as your personal Lord and Saviour! The Bible is quite clear!"

My heart sinks like a stone. I'm no fan of Mrs. Thatcher, but even less so of 'hell'. I'd stopped thinking about hell years ago. But this old-time sermon deeply unsettles me and doubts about my faith start to twist in my head like a knife. To be sure, Jesus himself appears to warn against hell in the Gospels. So I dig more deeply and read extensively about the biblical text on this matter. The scholarly consensus is that such words had probably been put into the mouth of Jesus by the gospel writers themselves who, after all, were writing several decades after his death and resurrection, with only 'oral tradition' to go on.

But while reading about this, I also notice that most scholars point out the contradictions in the various resurrection narratives—the very foundation of the Christian faith. I sort of 'knew' all this from my time at St John's but I didn't want to believe it. But now, ten years later, the door of doubt has been kicked firmly open again. Intuitively and depressingly, I sense that the sermon on hell is just the beginning—and God only knows where it will all end.

7. The Dark Night
1981–3

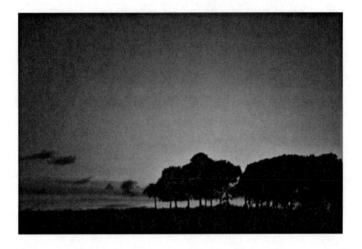

"It's bronchitis, Mr Adams, and you've got it quite bad. But here's a prescription that should improve things; you'll need to be off school for at least three weeks."

Healthwise, I've been lucky. Just the usual children's illnesses but nothing since then. But now I'm struggling with hot and cold sweats, constant coughing that brings up phlegm and with it, depression. I'm expecting the prescription to relieve these symptoms and it does—except for the depression. Instead, it becomes significantly worse.

To distract myself, I watch some daytime TV and I opt for a school programme on descriptive writing. In hindsight, it's a terrible choice. For the theme is *Hiroshima—the reflections of Japanese children*. As their heart-rending poems are read out (with subtitles), we are shown a film and photographs of what happened to human bodies during the blast and firestorm of the first atomic bomb. The images are terrifying, beyond description or belief. I want to turn away, but I cannot. I see it through.

From depression, I sink into a bottomless chasm, not only about what humans will do to each other, but why a so-called God of Love should ever permit it? Even allowing for human free will, God's omniscience would have foreseen it and his omnipotence could have stopped it—according to traditional Christian doctrines. Surely, a loving deity would not have created a world with such terrifying potential that he foreknew humans would abuse? Surely, this cannot be 'the best of all possible worlds'? Perhaps there's no God at all or if there is, then He's the Devil.

That day, my faith is stripped bare like the flesh of the Hiroshima victims, as my mind is wracked with 'the problem of evil'. But I cannot, and do not want to, give up on God as He is still the source of my life, my meaning, my love for Sophie and my vocation. Surely, there's an answer to this seemingly impossible riddle!

As I start to recover physically (but not mentally), I take myself off to various religious bookshops and buy whatever I can find about 'the problem of evil'. I consume these books, looking for an answer that will bring me some peace. Books with titles such as *Why Do Men Suffer? Evil and a God of Love. The Crucified God. The Theology of Auschwitz. The Pain that Heals. Cancer and a God of Love. The Passion of Man. Suffering.* And many others besides.

I also buy books about depression and *The Dark Night of the Soul*—a Catholic concept, not an evangelical one. On the occasions when I visit my parents, I have all these books stacked up by the sofa and I'm reading all the time. They don't know what's come over me and neither do I. I suffer from constant headaches and tiredness, and even John Hick's classic work on the subject [30], though impressive, fails to convince.

Perhaps, one day, I shall emerge from the darkness and experience God again and feel Him close. Perhaps I won't. And perhaps not knowing is part of the test, a pre-condition of the Dark Night. Meanwhile, I'm continually shifting in my religious self-identity. For I can no longer think of myself as a 'conservative evangelical'. So I try being a 'neo-orthodox' evangelical for a while. But *any* sort of evangelical is meant to be proclaiming the gospel of God's love from the rooftops—and it's a long time since I last did that. Now, it's more a case of hanging on to God by my fingernails because I *need* him to be there for me.

*

83

Eventually, exhausted from all my reading and with little to show for it, I conclude that searching for an answer to 'the problem of evil' is like looking for a needle in a haystack. Except the needle doesn't actually exist—it's just all haystack.

I'm still a Christian, but one who is unsure of so many things, so I'm coming to think of myself as a 'Christian Agnostic'. I can live with that, for the time being at least. And on that basis, I continue with my chaplaincy duties at school.

But nothing, it seems, is fixed. Everything is in flux.

All that once seemed solid is now melting into thin air [31].

8. The True Wilderness
1984–5

"Hi Jamie, so how's God these days?"

I mumble into my cornflakes and leave abruptly, my breakfast suddenly over. I later apologise to Miriam, a fellow Christian summer camp leader, without giving a reason for my churlish behaviour. Her innocent question has upset and alarmed me. I don't want to think about or admit that 'God' has gone AWOL from my life. I haven't talked to Him for ages, and He certainly hasn't talked to me, or perhaps I haven't been listening. Neither have I felt His presence recently. God is no longer a personal Friend and Saviour but merely the endpoint of a tortured theological argument, which I am finding increasingly difficult to sustain. My spiritual life has become an arid and desolate wasteland a sand-blown wilderness, a desert. It feels as though *The Hollow Men* from my teenage years have returned to haunt me.

*

Following the Christian summer camp, I start a day-release course in Nottingham about 'Community (World) Religions'. I need to attend this for my own religious integrity as well to support a broader-based RE curriculum at school. In the first two weeks, we join the worshippers of Krishna in a large and colourful Hindu temple and the devotees of Sai Baba in an inner-city house-temple. In the following weeks, we visit an Islamic Mosque, a Sikh Gurdwara, an Orthodox Synagogue, with a day-trip to a Buddhist monastery in the Lake District.

I'm certainly not about to convert to another religion, but I am made to think. What right do Christians have to claim superiority over these devoted worshippers and their sincerely held beliefs? Perhaps they are as much in contact with the divine as we are and compared with me, probably more so! I note the considerable similarities between all the religions, including Christianity, which leaves me wondering whether religion is just a cultural artefact that has been generated by societies in times of historic, social and cultural need. My belief in the uniqueness of Christianity feels under threat, and this coincides with my serious questioning of Christ's divinity. According to the scholarly consensus, Jesus was probably a radical Jewish prophet who (mistakenly) thought that the End of the World was nigh, and whose first followers (mistakenly) thought that he had risen from the dead and (mistakenly) exalted him to the status of the Incarnate Son of God. That's a lot of mistakes upon which to base one's faith.

I also have questions about the moral values of traditional Christianity—about pre-marital sex, abortion, divorce, homosexuality, euthanasia and women priests. I find myself in disagreement with the traditional Christian view on each of these matters. The foundations of my Christian landscape are moving, both externally and within. I'm struggling to hold on to my faith in a religious wilderness where the sand-dunes are continually shifting and reforming in the wind. Moreover, I'm struggling alone—unwilling to openly admit my continuing crisis to myself or to share it with Sophie and risk undermining her faith too.

*

At the conclusion of the Community Religions course, I pop into the nearby SPCK bookshop to search for a book about the relationship of Christianity to the other great world religions. Instead, I'm attracted to a slim volume of sermons: *The True Wilderness* by H. A. Williams. Originally published in 1965 [32], these unusual sermons were delivered by Harry Williams in the chapel of Trinity College, Cambridge, to mark his return to ministry after his own mental breakdown. His breakdown was primarily about his acceptance of his homosexuality in spite of the law (as it was then) and a hostile church. As part of his recovery, he fundamentally re-examined what the Christian faith and life were all about, through years of psychoanalysis and by absorbing the ideas of Sigmund Freud and Carl Jung.

The essence of his sermons is the importance of rediscovering oneself and of not repressing uncomfortable thoughts and feelings that arise from the unconscious, as we allow it to yield up its darker secrets. It means understanding the Christian faith in personal, psychological terms—not just the bare statements of Creed or Bible. Only by sacrificing our barren church orthodoxy might our souls be resurrected into becoming who we truly are, rather than who we might like, or pretend, ourselves to be [33].

I find it impossible to put the book down, as it seems to describe my own situation so accurately. Perhaps I am not so alone after all, for here is an Anglican minister who is giving me permission to accept myself with all my doubts and misgivings, yet not judging me for it. To the contrary, he claims this is 'the true wilderness' where we will rediscover ourselves and the *real* God—not the pretend God of hymns and prayers and sanctimonious religious chatter.

One passage I find especially apposite:

Most people's wilderness is inside them, not outside... Our wilderness then is an inner isolation. It's an absence of contact. It's a sense of being alone—boringly alone, or saddeningly alone, or terrifyingly alone... Or perhaps I've been robbed, robbed of my easy certainties, my unthinking convictions, that this is black and this is white...fantasies, like children's bricks out of which I thought I should build my life, and which have melted into the air, leaving me with nothing [34].

It would be difficult to find a better description of just how I am thinking and feeling right now.

*

After devouring *The True Wilderness*, I read his other books. In particular, *Tensions* illuminates an aspect of my life that I don't like, don't want to admit and haven't a clue what to do about. In recent years, I have come to feel worryingly immature, with the emotions and reactions of a child. I don't feel grown up at all and wonder what it must be like to be 'a man'. A bit of gentle teasing and a few moments of frustration have, in past months, sent me running upstairs in tears or driving the car idiotically and dangerously from pent-up anger—and I don't know why. *Tensions* provides me with a clue: according to Williams, *religion keeps us as dependent children*. It doesn't like us to grow up, arguing with and rebelling against God and standing on our own two feet. However:

Resentment, rebellion and self-assertion...is absolutely necessary if our relationship with God is to grow into maturity. And unless this is recognised, we shall...remain God's good little boys, futile and ineffective half-people [35].

I can recognise all of this in myself, but feel helpless what to do about it—like the child I am.

*

Having read all of Harry Williams' books that I can find, there still remain two troubling problems: 1. Harry Williams never seems to doubt God's existence. God is a 'given' for him. Whereas for me, this is at the very heart of my internal conflicts, so perhaps we are not quite on the same page after all. 2. I understand all the stuff about Freud, Jung, the unconscious and repression—and it's all very illuminating and helpful. But I don't see any *intrinsic* connection with Jesus and the Gospels, which feel like 'Christian extras'—interesting, but not essential. For me, it's the gospel according to Freud that is the distilled essence of Williams' sermons and writings.

But, if that is the case, why am I still hankering after God and Jesus?

9. The Shipwreck

1985–6

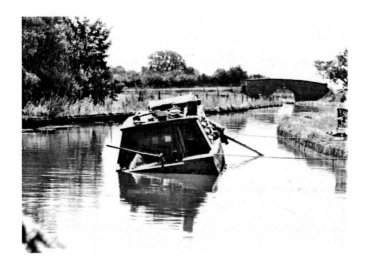

The shipwreck—both real and also symbolic.

As our hire-boat rounds a bend of the Oxford Canal, a sad and disconcerting sight comes into view—a private narrowboat, half-submerged and listing badly. Two gangplanks extend to the towpath as its occupants try to salvage what they can. One can only feel sympathy for them; someone's journey or grand adventure gone desperately wrong, holed beneath the waterline—a poignant reminder of my own ship of faith, which had been similarly damaged by the Hiroshima film several years ago and has been letting on water ever since.

I've now relinquished the evangelical summer camps due to my disturbed and declining faith. But I've organised instead a narrowboat holiday for a group of Christian friends, including Miriam and Mike, two of my former camp leaders. None of them know about the parlous state of my own religious voyage, though I had given a few hints to a couple of those closest to me.

We slowly inch past the stricken vessel and thereafter, our cruise is trouble-free, apart from what continues to go on inside my head. I get some light relief from my inner torment, due to the endless hours of sun, the flowing wine and the joy of navigating a seventy-foot narrowboat through the winding course of England's canal system.

*

As our journey's end approaches, we all agree that an informal communion service would be a fitting conclusion to the week. As I am the only ordained minister on board, it falls to me to officiate. I feel that I cannot preach from the Bible as it has lost all meaning for me, so I preach from Harry Williams' writings and, I suspect, a few eyebrows are raised.

After the service, Mike makes a speech thanking people for their various contributions to the week's enjoyment. Gwen gets thanked for making a cooked breakfast each day. Ben gets thanked for providing all the wine, and so on. Virtually, everyone gets a mention; everyone that is, except me, who had organised the holiday from beginning to end, sorted out the various finances and had consulted everyone from start to finish. As the formalities come to an end, people start to chat and play music, but I remain silent and disconsolate. This omission of any gratitude towards me feels like a punch in the stomach that I hadn't seen coming, but what am I to do? I feel like shouting and screaming like a two-year-old who's persistently ignored by their parents, but to do this would mean a public meltdown, and I'm not prepared for that, with all of its consequences.

Without talking to anyone, I walk off into the night along the towpath, my hurt feelings tumbling continuously until they can fall no further. My despair is not primarily about the slight from Mike (though that is bad enough), but it's about my utterly immature reaction of not being able to cope with it. I realise that I don't have the adult resources to deal with the situation as I'm so desperately in need for recognition and affirmation. Neither have I any religious resources to turn to, for they have long since disappeared.

I walk for an hour and although it's starting to get cold, I decide to stick it out until midnight, giving me an hour-and-a-half walk back. I want them to miss me, even to worry about me and to wonder what might have triggered off my lengthy disappearance. When I return, only Ben and Miriam are waiting up for me and they ask me if I'm okay.

"Crap!" is my single-word response as I head for my bunk and long for morning.

When morning finally arrives, I accept the cup of tea on offer, but I speak to no one. I then head for the back of the boat for some solo steering until we arrive back at the boatyard. There, the rest of the crew take group photos and embrace each other before parting. But I'm having none of it. I just shout a terse "I'm off!", then climb into my car for some solitude and relief. During the drive home, I wonder what I'm going to say to Sophie and how I'm going to cope with the morning service the following day, which I had previously agreed to take for a local vicar.

I simply tell Sophie that the canal holiday was "crap" and that I don't want to talk about it; our relationship is in a delicate state as well as my faith and my emotional immaturity. At the church service the following day, I put on my best Christian face and get through the ordeal intact. But as I walk back to my car deep in thought, I make a momentous decision: *I can't go on like this anymore.*

*

I decide to resign my Anglican Orders. I am not emotionally fit to be a minister and any remaining faith that I have is not worth sharing with anyone. It may also mean resigning from my school post, but I will cross that bridge when I come to it. Back at the flat, I inform Sophie of my decision, but I am not willing to discuss it. It's too fresh, too raw, too difficult and too embarrassing.

When the autumn term starts, I meet with the Head and he is generous to a fault. He himself is an ordained Anglican minister (of a liberal outlook) and he agrees to take upon himself some of my chaplaincy duties, while farming the rest out to local ministers. So long as I can continue with my full timetable of RE teaching, my pay won't be affected. I am touched by his kindness and concern. He hopes that I will find a way through my current problems but I just can't see it; my doubts seem all-consuming. So I struggle on... I am able to teach, but I just can't believe.

*

Six months later, I hand in my resignation from my school post. The great ship of faith, which has kept my life afloat for almost two decades, finally disappears into the deep, dragging my long-term relationship with Sophie with it (3.4). By the end of my final term, I have already left my home with Sophie, and have moved into a back-to-back terrace.

I decide to write an open letter to all my friends—all of them Christians—setting out what I can of the reasons for my loss of faith, my resignation of Anglican Orders and my failed relationship with Sophie. In it, I attach no blame to anyone but myself and my circumstances. I send out fifty letters and I'm curious about what sort of replies I might receive: empathetic? consoling? supportive? intrigued? or of judgement, in the name of evangelical religion? I needn't have worried, for I receive not a single reply, ever. Neither does anyone phone or call to see me except Mike, who apologises for his oversight on the boat. I am shattered by how quickly all but one of my so-called Christian friends have deserted me. It is further evidence for my private theory that the more traditionally religious people are, the less humane they are likely to be. And the more liberal or non-religious people are, the more likely they are to act in a kind and caring way.

Thankfully, my school community is far more humane and generous than my deserting religious friends. At my farewell assembly, I speak to the gathering of staff and students, not with a text from the Bible, nor even from Harry Williams, but with a skit from Rowan Atkinson:

Where are we? How did we get here? Why did we come? Where do we want to go? How do we want to get to where we want to go? How far do we have to go before we get to where we want to be? How would we know where we were when we got there? Have we got a map? [36].

The whole school assembly is in hysterics as I play the original sketch in its entirety. I then proffer a few words of wisdom, suggesting that the best map we have to guide us through life's course is learning to be true to ourselves—a familiar theme of Harry Williams. Of course, the skit is great fun and is primarily aimed at myself, but I hope it interests as well as amuses a few others. I don't think God gets a mention.

And then, all too soon it's: "Thank you all, and goodbye" as the assembly erupts with cheers and loud applause. I'm both touched and taken aback, even though I've already received, from both staff and students, many 'thank you' cards, gifts and warm wishes for my future.

*

But what future?

Even as I'm drinking in the applause and receiving hugs and handshakes from the departing assembly, I'm acutely aware that my life is about to change beyond all recognition—and not in a good way.

For, with a shipwrecked faith, a failed relationship, no job and deserting friends, I have nothing to motivate me and nowhere to go, except a back-to-back terrace in a dead-end street—my own Desolation Row [37].

10. Religious Crises: Review
1964–86

i.   From the age of nine, my life was marked by my passionate support for Coventry City—an attachment to an institution—which substituted for, and superimposed itself upon my insecure and ambivalent attachment to my parents. My attachment to my parents is primary and probably hard-wired into my brain from my early formative years [38]. The reason why Coventry City became an attachment figure for me was probably because it was reliable (being an institution) and because, for fans like me, it provided an outlet for emotional expression, unlike my controlling parents.

ii.   It felt strange that my intense feelings of emptiness first occurred in the midst of my football euphoria. However, it may simply be that: *Sadness naturally accompanies the recognition that an attachment figure is not accessible* [39]; on that day, the attachment figure of Coventry City simply wasn't available to me in the way and with the intensity I wanted (see 2.1). Studies by Weiss and others suggest that feelings of loneliness and of being 'silent, dead, empty or hollow' are common characteristics of those who are insecurely and anxious-ambivalently attached [40].

iii.   It was also unexpected that at the very height of the *Sky Blue Revolution* in 1967, I decide to detach myself from Coventry City and fully attach myself to evangelical Christianity instead. Many people support their football team *and* follow their religion at the same time. There was a short period (Sept 1966-7) when both co-existed in my life. So why did evangelical religion eventually win out? Because it met more of my attachment needs than did Coventry City, because it was *personal* in a way that Coventry City wasn't, and in three ways: 1. Jesus was my personal Friend and Saviour, with whom I had a personal connection and to whom I could talk [41]. 2. Through the local churches, there was a much richer social life for me, including girls. 3. In April 1967, I started going out with Celia and soon realised that Saturday afternoons would be far more enjoyable snuggled up with her on her sofa than shivering on a hard seat in a football stand.

iv.   Evangelical Christianity was then an improved substitute attachment. Although this too was an institutional attachment, the personal element was very strong. *God can be regarded as demonstrating all the defining features of an attachment figure*, as Lee Kirkpatrick, an attachment researcher, points out [42]. As a bonus, evangelical Christianity also offered two further elements that were appealing to an A-level student in the middle of the Cold War: firstly, an intellectual stimulus for a reflective teenage mind, for example, T. S. Eliot (2.2) and the Bible, and also hope in the face of catastrophe, nuclear or otherwise (1.8), through its offering of eternal life to all those who believe [43].

v.   Further considerations include Freud's view that adolescent religious conversion is merely the replacement of human parents by an 'Almighty Father' as one was transiting from childhood to adulthood. More pertinent to me is James Marcia's view that adolescent crises vary [44], and that I may have experienced a crisis of *identity foreclosure*. In other words, I made a hasty decision to commit to evangelical Christianity without having properly weighed up all the pros and cons of this and other possible routes through adolescence. Those who are anxiously attached (like me) are more likely to throw themselves headlong into a new identity (2.3) to avoid the anxiety of waiting—not knowing what the future will hold. An understanding of such rash and impulsive behaviour has recently been gained by research into the prefrontal cortex, which is the final brain region to fully mature—'not going fully online until the mid-twenties' [45]. As a consequence, an adolescent or young adult may "transform physics, have hideous fashion taste, break their neck recreationally or commit their life to God" [46]. Or, as I did, smuggle Bibles through the Berlin Wall, aspire to be the next Billy

Graham and give away all my pop records to charity (2.3), as well as commit my life to God!

vi.   Credence must also be given to Kirkpatrick's extensive research in this field, using, as he does, the meta-studies of others as well as his own. His conclusion is that anxious-insecure individuals find in God *the kind of attachment relationship that has been missing from their interpersonal relationships. When this occurs, 'falling in love' with God tends to occur rapidly and dramatically, leading at least sometimes to a sudden religious conversion* [47]. Such conversions are more likely during adolescence than at any other time [48]. It would seem then, that there is a triple vulnerability factor at work towards religious conversion for anxious-ambivalently attached teenagers, such as myself. a. Because they have an anxious-insecure attachment to their parents. b. Because they are transiting the unstable period from childhood to adulthood. c. Because of their immature prefrontal cortex.

It is perhaps not too surprising then that about twenty of my sixth-form friends went through a similar religious experience to me (and perhaps through my influence), although only two of us went the whole hog and entered into the ordained ministry.

vii.   At the *Battle for the Mind* lecture in Durham (2.4), it seems that I suddenly discovered my prefrontal cortex! It was the first time I had done any rational thinking about my faith, apart from deciding whether St Paul had meant this or that or something else by a particular text. But my post-lecture logical conclusions threw me into violent conflict with my faith as an emotional attachment, leaving me with perpetual *cognitive dissonance*, i.e., mental stress caused by holding two contradictory beliefs at the same time or by encountering information that contradicts existing belief. Emotionally, I suffered extreme *separation-anxiety* from my divine attachment figure. In my agony of cognitive dissonance and anxious doubt, by far the strongest pull was from my emotional attachment to my faith, as upon it rested my whole identity, my meaning and my future life and career.

viii.   Therefore, my 'battle' to restore my faith through 'proxy faith', scholarship and Francis Schaeffer (2.5) was, in attachment terms, an exercise of *proximity maintenance* towards my divine attachment figure. As God seemed to be in hiding (or was even possibly 'dead'), I had to work exceedingly hard to try to find Him again, like a distraught child in a huge department store looking for parents who are nowhere to be seen.

ix.   Thereafter, all my further training and ministry was conducted in the searchlight of *chronic vigilance*—on the lookout for anything that could disturb my shaky faith: a possible mistake in the Bible perhaps? Or news of an earthquake or other natural disaster that would trigger off serious doubts about an omnipotent and loving God (2.7). After such news-media tragedies, it would take me several days before I could recover any sort of equilibrium. I was like a lover who is continually on the lookout for signs of unfaithfulness in their beloved, and often thinks they have found some. Recovery from such threats is neither comfortable, quick nor easy, as one is continually anxious.

x.   With a great deal of hindsight, it seems that myself and Christianity were not a well-suited couple. It was only for a relatively brief period that God was my *secure base* [49] for evangelism, ministry and Christian summer camps (2.3). Dr Sargant's lecture had taught me that spiritual experiences couldn't be relied upon and now, given the 'problems' of Hell and Evil (2.6 and 2.7), God did not seem to be very reliable either. My belief in Biblical inerrancy was, for a time, an important bulwark against doubt [50], but when that also became untenable (2.6), all I could do was cling to God as a *safe haven* amid the gathering storm. In other words, my attachment needs remained strong, even if my attachment object was disappearing into the ether.

xi.   The basic attachment function of religion as a safe haven also started to feel redundant, as my lack of self-knowledge (2.8) and emotional immaturity (2.9) became increasingly apparent. With my faith shipwrecked, I became detached from my illusory attachment figure and withdrew from all forms of religion (2.9). Kirkpatrick cites several studies that suggest that *problematic childhood relationships with parents are also associated with an increased likelihood of de-conversion from religion in adulthood* [51]. To summarise, anxious and ambivalent individuals like me tend to be unstable and are therefore more prone to both religious conversion *and* de-conversion [52].

xii.   I now believe that my major religious crisis of de-conversion was in fact the expression of a delayed adolescent crisis along the lines suggested by Erik Erikson [53]. Evangelical religion had maintained my childhood dependencies and identity foreclosure had prevented me from achieving an independent adolescent identity. The start of my psychological adulthood therefore coincided with my de-conversion from religion—I had a lot of catching up to do for me to become and feel like a man.

Summary:

1. My religious conversion was the product of an insecure childhood and ambivalent attachment status, combined with an adolescent crisis and immature prefrontal cortex.

2. My religious de-conversion was the product of an insecure childhood and an anxious-ambivalent attachment status, combined with a developmental need to 'grow up', both cognitively and emotionally.

3. Whether either or both of these major crises (religious conversion and de-conversion) should be viewed positively, negatively or neutrally is open to debate. It seems to me that there are positive, regrettable and neutral elements in each.

4. At the time, it certainly felt that the conversion was very positive and the de-conversion extremely negative, but today I view this the other way round.

5. My major crisis of religious de-conversion was, in fact, a delayed adolescent crisis, as I had not achieved an independent adolescent identity during adolescence itself.

6. The extensive research of Lee Kirkpatrick and others demonstrate that there are many links between religious beliefs and commitment, and attachment needs and behaviours, including the processes of religious

conversion, de-conversion and acute separation-anxiety when faith is lost.

*

To support positive mental health:

As adolescents, it's wise not to over-commit to any person or cause without plenty of rational reflection taking place first. It's also better for one's mental health to review as many options as possible, consulting with wise peers and adults along the way. Listen out for any warning signs of extreme emotions or erratic behaviour and be prepared to ask yourself—and others—'what's this all about?' Be honest with yourself and with any confidantes about what's concerning you before deciding too quickly about your future. Simply acting on an ill-thought out impulse may lead you to have regrets later on, or even to a later crisis or breakdown. Finally, beware of any groups or organisations that try to rush you into immediate commitment to a cause—be it religious, political, financial or charitable. It's YOUR life, so don't throw it away. Look before you leap.

Chapter 3 ~ Romantic Passions

1967–93

1. In Dreams
(Roy Orbison, 1963)
April 1967

I'm in Dreamland! At least, I hope and indeed expect to be, tonight!

There's a girl at the Baptist youth club, Celia, who I really like and, on the bus this morning, her cousin told me that she really likes me too! So tonight's the night for asking her out, but only after the youth club has finished, as I'm not risking a public rejection. Perhaps Lady Luck will smile on me at last, or perhaps I should say 'God willing', having now been a 'born-again' Christian for over a year.

*

As the youth club is finishing, I grab my coat and leave, hoping that Celia will follow me, alone. We've spent most of the evening together but I'm still pretty nervous and waiting for her to leave seems like eternity. Perhaps she's stopped to chat. Eventually, the door opens and out she steps, by herself. So far, so good, as I step out from the shadows and into her path.

"Hello again! Can I walk home with you?"

"Of course, you can, but it's two miles and then you'll have to come all the way back…"

We walk on, a few feet apart, in an awkward silence until I can stand it no longer and just spit it out.

"Your cousin had a word with me this morning. So, will you go out with me? As my girlfriend?"

She laughed: "Of course I will! I thought you'd never ask!"

Heaving a huge sigh of relief and hardly being able to believe my ears, we immediately slipped our arms around each other, and there they remained. When we eventually reached her front gate, she took me by the hand and led me onto the front porch where we started, and continued, kissing for half an hour or more. Such relief! Such sweet kisses! I was in Dreamland at last—but a very real dreamland too! After so many teenage years longing for a proper girlfriend, I'm now with the loveliest girl in the world! She's slim, blonde and bubbly—the very nicest person I've ever met!

*

While we're still on the porch, her father opens the front door and is very welcoming: "In future, bring the lad in and you can use the front room—we shan't interrupt you."

Celia also asks me if I'd like to see her the following Saturday afternoon, which I would. But there's a problem! It's *Coventry City v Wolverhampton Wanderers* at Highfield Road—the most important game in City's 84-year history and on the brink of promotion to the First Division for the very first time. With divided loyalties, I decline her invitation, hoping it doesn't put her off, but I needn't have worried. City win and get promoted so I'm in triple dreamland now—with Celia, City and God!

We enjoy a few months of bliss, then I'm off to Berlin with the Coventry diocese and, shortly afterwards, Celia goes off to Switzerland with the Baptist church youth fellowship. We write every day—she's everything I could wish for in a girlfriend. When the football season restarts, I decide not to renew my season ticket, preferring to spend Saturday afternoons and evenings with Celia, going out for walks or, as winter approaches, lapping up her affection in her front room. Having felt starved of affection all my life, I can't get enough of it, and neither can she, it seems. Sometimes we study the Bible together, mainly St Paul, as he seems much more evangelical than Jesus! We also listen to two LPs over and over again: Billy Graham's *London Crusade Choir* and Jim Reeves' *Gospel Songs*—and that's as 'pop' as it gets!

The following year, we both go on the Baptist youth holiday to Switzerland where we're able to slip away most nights for some more intimate times together. I become very aroused, and that's how it stays for the rest of the holiday, quite painful at times, but I don't let on. There's another problem—sex before marriage is completely prohibited in the evangelical way of life. We know that we can never complete what we start, which is very frustrating. We go so far then we have to backtrack to the earlier stages, before starting all over again. We both remain strong and in complete agreement, despite the inconvenience.

However, our circumstances soon change as, after a year together, I go away to St John's College, Durham, while Celia continues her normal routine of home, work and church. We are apart for eight weeks at a time, with only daily letters and the occasional phone call. After the *Battle for the Mind* lecture (2.4), I'm in a quandary. I would like to share everything with her. But I don't feel I can share *this* with her because: 1. I don't want to admit my faith problems, even to myself. 2. I don't want to risk undermining Celia's own belief, as she prides herself on her 'simple' unquestioning faith. 3. If my doubts persist, I don't want to risk Celia breaking up with me. I need her love and affection more than ever—she's all I've got! So I don't tell her about the lecture and its effect on me, although I do indicate that some aspects of my theology degree are quite complicated.

*

In the summer term, my parents bring Celia up to Durham for the weekend. I have a surprise for her when she visits me in my college room. I propose, and she immediately and gleefully accepts! We agree to get married as soon as I finish at St John's in two years' time. Throughout the year, we continually plan the wedding and our friends back in Coventry are delighted for us. They've been expecting it and think we're exceedingly well-matched. They can't see us ever breaking up.

Due to the emotional security provided by our engagement and since I've come across the writings of Francis Schaeffer (2.5), I'm feeling more hopeful that I shall get through my crisis of faith and come out stronger on the other side. But as Celia visits me for a second time at St John's, I get a subliminal feeling that a large cultural gap exists between us, that mentally, we are living in different worlds. Physically however, we get even closer to each other, possibly to compensate for the unspoken fear of a growing personal and cultural distance.

During the summer, we holiday together at a Christian-run hotel in Cornwall. Celia spends her time 'fellowshipping' with the other Christian guests, whereas I'm more interested in the Five Points of Calvinism [54] about which a fellow guest has recently written a thesis—and I discuss this at length with him. But it's not something I talk to Celia about as I can't imagine her being interested in T.U.L.I.P.: i.e., **T**otal depravity; **U**nconditional election; **L**imited atonement;

Irresistible grace; and the **P**erseverance of the saints—I can't think why! But to me, it's the very essence of my new 'Reformed' faith. The holiday is otherwise good and enjoyable (apart from the sexual prohibitions) and I start my third year at Durham with high hopes for my faith, our love and, before long, our married life together.

*

However, what I had conveniently forgotten from my previous (although brief) romantic encounters is that although romantic dreams can be wonderful, especially if they become reality, they do have the unfortunate habit of coming to an end—when a loud alarm clock goes off and you are suddenly returned to the single life from whence you came.

2. It's Over
(Roy Orbison, 1964)
1970-1

It's evening in mid-December as, tense and excited, I peer down my road, lit by yellow streetlamps and multicoloured Christmas displays. I've just returned from Durham and, right on time as usual, I see Celia turn the corner and walk briskly up the road to our front gate. After six long weeks apart, I'm so looking forward to being back in her arms and tasting her sweet kisses again! Now that my faith is almost restored, I'm feeling more positive than for many months and looking forward to further planning for our wedding in just over six months' time! I wave to her from my room, but she's not looking… I open the front door with glee, whereupon she gives me a brief hug, says a quick 'hi' to my parents and then races upstairs to my room. Her abruptness is unusual.

*

She sits at the end of the bed looking downcast but saying nothing, before starting to cry. She cries continuously for several minutes—with me at a loss—until she is drained of tears. I'm in shock; in almost four years together, I've never seen her cry before. Perhaps her mother is terminally ill or some other great tragedy has happened. It's all of five minutes, though it feels like an hour to me, before she manages enough composure for one chilling sentence.

"Jamie, I'm very, very, sorry, but I don't love you anymore and I can't marry you."

With that, she takes off her engagement ring and places it on the coffee table between us. Within a few minutes, she's gone, leaving me shattered and bewildered. She offers no further explanation and I am too shocked to ask for one. Later, I learn that my parents went to visit Celia's parents to see if there was anything that could be done, but apparently not. The only information they gleaned is that Celia thought I was too 'brainy' for her—her self-deprecating way of saying that there was indeed a significant difference between our worlds and that, during my time at Durham, I had changed from being the outgoing evangelical convert she had fallen in love with to the preoccupied and tortured soul I had become.

I was back from St John's to celebrate my twenty-first birthday and then Christmas—together with Celia. As for my birthday party, I proceed with it, but without her. It's an awkward and dour affair as my friends, all in couples, are also in a state of shock. I stumble through Christmas in a twilight zone, expressing my anguish to God in daily prayer, which seems to help. Then one of my friends declares that he has received a 'prophecy' from God, telling him that Celia and I will soon be reunited. I am disturbed by this, wanting to believe it so very much, but I'm unwilling to trust any claims for 'spiritual experiences', especially in the light of the Sargant lecture. Unsurprisingly, my friend's 'prophecy' proves false—and I'm still waiting for his apology.

So, in just under two years, I've been on the receiving end of two massive shocks, neither of which I had any inkling of beforehand. I've been hit by the proverbial London bus that I didn't know was there—two of them!

*

I'm concerned how the end of my precious relationship with Celia will affect my studies and preparation for finals in six months' time. But I needn't worry for, back at St John's, the pain of loss is eased by familiar surroundings and my college friends. My faith is gradually being restored and I can devote myself fully to all my studies, including my self-chosen extra-curricular work in Christian apologetics and systematic theology.

A few months later, I receive a pleasant surprise from some of the female students at the Christian Union. It's time for the May College Balls, and they don't want me to miss out just because I don't have a partner. So they arrange for a friend of theirs (whose boyfriend is globe-trotting) to accompany me to the St John's and St Mary's balls—and to play some tennis as well. To prepare for the dances, I buy a new *Beach Boys* LP and try out some dance moves—a timely reminder that I'm single again and free to date single Christian girls [55]. I enjoy the college balls, but less so the tennis, as I'm thoroughly beaten by the captain of the University women's first team, as I later discover. Still, I have enjoyed my brief foray back into the pop and girly world of my teenage years. It's a welcome dose of fresh air.

Finals go well and I gain a good 2:1 degree, with my tutor suggesting that I should consider doing a Master's degree. My parents are proud to see me graduate. Of my problems with Celia, they were, more or less, fully aware. But of my trials of faith, they knew absolutely nothing, except what they might have gathered from my piles of serious reading and my depressed mood whenever I visited them for weekends.

*

That summer at home, I meet up with church friends, most of whom who are also returning from university. Cleo had just graduated with a degree in Japanese and on a couple of occasions, we meet up to chat and share our university experiences—but it's not long before we're sharing more than our thoughts. It's good to feel such affection and desire again—six months after Celia had broken up with me—although, frustratingly, Cleo and I continue to uphold the strict evangelical prohibition on sex. We meet for two such evenings and then she's off to Japan—and that's the last I see of her.

After three long years at Durham, I'm a survivor, just, from two separate, massive shocks: a shocked and broken faith following the Sargant lecture, and a shocked romance and broken engagement brought about by Celia's sudden departure. Having survived both of these, what I hope for now is a doubt-free faith and ministry, and a reliable romance and marriage—until death do us part.

So, my first big romance has come to a shattering end after almost four years together.

But I soon find myself wondering whether such love will come around for me, again.

3. The Eyes Have It
1973-6

She catches me by surprise—as she eyes me from the bed in the corner of her room, where a dozen or so undergraduates are gathered. Every time I glance in her direction, her gaze meets mine with increasing intensity. Her hazel eyes stay focussed on me and I feel that everyone in the room is watching, for I'd never been on the receiving end of such blatant flirtation before.

*

I'm at Cambridge doing my theology MA. After attending the Christian Union's main Saturday evening lecture, I'm invited to one of the after-meeting coffee parties taking place in a college next door to mine. Such parties consist mainly of music, coffee and chat as we sit or crouch on every available piece of furniture or floor in Holly's room. After a somewhat heated debate about the evening's talk, the mood lightens and I catch Holly's eyes firmly focussed on mine. This happens several times, so I'm convinced that she's interested in me. But, unsure of how to respond, I exit the scene in a fluster—and only return as the rest are leaving. Holly pats the space beside her on the bed and I waste no time in joining her, as we wait, impatiently, for the room to finally clear.

We politely confirm our names and the courses we are on: theology for me and history for her. We talk for half an hour about this and that, knowing there's a hidden sexual agenda. Then suddenly, we cease talking as our mouths make for each other and become locked. Buttons are undone and T-shirts teased out, before we both pull away and sit bolt upright, tucking ourselves in to conceal our embarrassment.

"I think we're going too fast! No sex before marriage and all that!" Holly proclaims as we return to interspersed talking and kissing. I agree. Nevertheless, later that night, as I climb the fence that separates Holly's college from mine,

I'm elated by the physical contact I've just enjoyed and by the new relationship that I assume has just started. Next day, I miss early morning chapel, preferring to lie in bed and think unholy thoughts about Holly, whom I'll be seeing later that evening.

*

This is my first proper date with Holly and is very different from the previous night. I've been invited for a meal with her next-door neighbours, which they have cooked up together in the communal kitchen. Afterwards, we spend some time chatting over coffee in Ella's room. I suspect that Holly wants her friends to give me the once-over but I don't mind their questioning as they are both attractive, well-spoken girls. Later, Holly and I return to her room, now strangely quiet after the previous night's events. Pretty quickly, we get physical again, but in a more restrained way, and I leave before midnight as we both have early Monday morning lectures.

As I leave, I can see Holly's nose pressed against her window as she waves goodbye until I'm out of sight. As I climb the fence back to my college, my feelings are different this time. I have a feeling of unease and discomfort in the pit of my stomach but I don't know why, except that I simply don't have the feelings for Holly that I *still* have for Celia. I'm not in love with Holly—perhaps, after Celia, I'll never be able to love anyone else! Perhaps, romantically speaking, I'm scarred for life!

Despite my emotional reservations, it soon becomes clear to me that Holly is very keen so I'm determined not to pass up lightly this new opportunity for love. Moreover, I'd been made very welcome by her friends. So I ignore my unease and it gradually fades, as we settle into a regular student relationship—but without the sex. Most of the time, I see Holly at her college—lunching together, playing squash or listening to music. I introduce her to my own college friends and she seems accepted there too.

As the weeks slip by, however, I start to notice that Holly seems to present a different persona at different times. At my college, or if we're going out, she dresses sharp, with short skirts to show off her slim figure and lovely legs. She wears make-up and heels and sways from the hips. She has the look and confidence of a model. When she adopts this persona, I think of her as *Holly, 1st class*; though, of course, I don't tell her that. At other times, however, she appears very different. No make-up or heels, just crumpled corduroys and trainers, her black hair tied back and slouching as she walks—*Holly, 2nd class*.

When she's *Holly 2nd class*, she appears to have a chip on her shoulder about something or other, as she's always putting other students down and sometimes herself. Over the summer, I stay with her for a week at her Sheffield home and realise that it might be to do with her working-class background, as she compares herself unfavourably to the privileged backgrounds of many Cambridge students.

I don't really mind Holly's dual personality (as I see it), except I'm never quite sure which one will turn up for any given date. I much prefer *Holly 1st class*, but I suspect this is more of a performance than *Holly 2nd class*. Perhaps she's sensed this and is colluding with my preferences while in Cambridge, in order to help the relationship along. But when staying with her in the summer, *Holly 1st class* all but disappears and I feel less attracted by her truer and more honest self.

Again, it seems that she's sensed this, because on the last day of my time in Sheffield, she surprises me with a change of sleeping arrangements. We'll be staying overnight with some married friends of hers who will be leaving for work first thing in the morning. I think nothing of it until, as soon as her friends leave, she appears in my room, leaning against the door in only a thin T-shirt and a thong. She looks at me with those doe-eyes of hers, that recall our very first meeting:

"Get up, lazy-bones, and come with me! While the cat's away, the mice can play!"

She grabs me by the hand and pulls me out of bed and into her bedroom: "Okay, no full sex but there's lots of interesting stuff we can do!"

Sitting on the bed, she invites me to lift off her T-shirt, which I do.

"Now it's my turn," as she pulls down my boxers—and stares.

"Well, you seem pleased to see me!" she quips, before disappearing under the sheets. There, we spend an exhilarating hour, getting ourselves entangled and disentangled—but without going the whole way.

*

And then, over breakfast, another surprise as she makes an announcement:

"I've been accepted to do a PhD at Newcastle. It's about traditional Christianity and radical socialism, with special reference to George Lansbury, the Labour Party leader in the 1930s. It will mean a long-distance relationship I'm afraid. I'm sorry, but it's something I really want to do."

I'm stunned by her news, though fascinated by her chosen subject.

While Holly is starting in Newcastle, I'm being ordained into the Anglican church and starting life in a Lincolnshire parish. Despite being 150 miles apart, we continue to see each other, but mainly at her end. As the months pass by, our meetings feel less satisfactory, and not only through sexual frustration. Although we're both evangelical Christians, Holly is getting more and more involved in radical left-wing politics at the university. While I try to be supportive, I'm certainly no socialist so we just don't see eye to eye about her political agenda. As a consequence, heated debates start to become a regular feature of my visits.

Sometimes she will cancel a visit at short notice because there's a rally or protest going on. She's also made her ambition quite clear—to become a researcher for the Labour Party in London, or even to enter the House of Commons as an MP. Yes, I can imagine that those eyes of hers could win her a whole load of votes!

The journeys to Newcastle seem to get longer as our times together become shorter and less satisfying. We're living in different worlds: I'm serving God in a rural Lincolnshire parish, but she's in academia preaching radical politics. Therefore, after a difficult relationship over several frustrating years, we decide to call it a day.

*

Several years later, I hear on the grapevine that Holly did indeed move to London and now works for the Labour Party inside the House of Commons, where *The Ayes Have It*—and, I imagine, her *Eyes Have It*, too.

As for me, I'm starting to eye up a different sort of life.

4. In a Spin
1976–85

"Morning, James. We're a small group this year—just three of us, in fact: myself, you and a young lady called Sophie, who should be here in a minute. There won't be any formal lectures, just a three-hour tutorial each week. I hope that's okay?"

*

Parish life hasn't suited me, apart from the church schools which I've enjoyed and which have given me an idea for a career change—teaching RE! It's my first day at a Teacher Training College near Lincoln and I'm a bit surprised—even disappointed—that the class is so small. The tutor is youngish and seems friendly. A young lady in her early twenties appears at the door and Sophie is formally introduced to me. There's a sharp intake of breath as Sophie is stunningly beautiful and I can feel myself going red in the neck as we politely shake hands. She sits down in the armchair next to me and it's difficult not to be drawn to her cascading blonde curls, which only partially obscures her cleavage that presses against her white, lacy blouse. It's difficult not to notice how, as she crosses her legs, her tight black skirt rises up to reveal a long and sensuous thigh.

Somehow, I manage to snap myself back to reality and focus on the course we're both starting, but I retain little of what the tutor says, except that he'll take us both to the bar afterwards and buy us a drink, which he does. After downing his pint and while I'm still eying up Sophie, he is up and off; with a twinkle in his eye: "I'll leave you two to get to know each other. Have fun!"

We both warm to his informal manner and sense of humour as we chat easily together and get ourselves another drink.

*

It turns out that we're both evangelical Christians, so there's a good rapport from the start. Later in the term, for my birthday, I invite her round to my flat and she arrives with a bottle and a birthday card—and a beaming smile! But we also discover a difference: she calls herself a *liberal evangelical*, which for her means that the Bible should be re-interpreted for the modern world. In other words, women's equality and being gay is okay, as is sex before marriage for couples who are engaged—and dressing sexily, of course! But I'm a *conservative evangelical* and I'm still working on these issues, although I'm less 'hard-line' than I used to be. I try to convince her that the Bible is infallible and contains no errors of fact, but she can't agree. After Christmas, we go to different schools for teaching practice and we lose touch with each other. I rather think that I've pushed her away.

When we meet again for a tutorial just before Easter, Sophie has problems, especially with her mother, which she tells me about. She asks me to help her move out of her mother's house, while she's away. However, when I arrive, she seems in no particular rush and sits me down for tea and scones by an open fire. Leonard Cohen is singing hauntingly in the background as Sophie invites me to join her on the sofa and starts flirting with me. I suddenly find myself in a very non-religious mood and I'm wondering if she wants to take things further. I soon find out.

"Jamie, let's go up to my bedroom then."

I follow her up the staircase, appreciating her perfect backside in her tight new jeans and wondering what's coming next. Once in the room, she switches on the light—a single lightbulb without a shade. There are a dozen cardboard boxes, all taped up and stacked in a corner.

"Here are the boxes I was telling you about," she says with a twinkle in her eye. "Are you okay with the large ones, and I'll bring the rest? I hope they'll all fit in your car!"

I'm suddenly deflated but we continue with the task in hand and get her moved out and into her new flat a few miles away. As I'm leaving, she gives me a hug and kisses me on both cheeks:

"Now off you go, but come back on Saturday and I'll cook tea for you, to say thank you."

*

When I arrive on Saturday, Sophie is looking her flirty and sexy best. I wonder if she's cooking up something else apart from tea. She is—she wants a heart-to-heart.

"Jamie, I know I tease you, it's because I really like you. I think we've got a bond, a connection. But you ought to know, in case you're wondering, I can never marry you."

Sophie is racing way ahead of me and I'm struggling to catch up. I'm elated that she seems to like me, but then surprised that she can't marry me—and I've not even proposed! Or even thought about it! My head's in a spin! Still, I appreciate her openness and honesty.

"Jamie, it's not you, it's me! I won't *ever* marry, because my parents' marriage is so horrific that I'm never going to take the same risk for myself—ever!"

I have to pinch myself that I'm even having this conversation, but we talk on into the early hours and agree that, for the time being, we just be boyfriend and girlfriend and see how it goes. We snuggle up on her sofa to kiss and cuddle—but I'm very careful to go no further. I don't want to end up in another long drawn-out and frustrating relationship, like I had with Holly. In any case, I want to be married and have a proper family, and Sophie's not available for that, so it would seem.

It starts to get light outside, so I make my way home, both elated and depressed at the same time. But then, within a few months, circumstances intervene and our situation shifts up a gear.

*

I'm on my way home from Leicester, from a job interview with the Inter-varsity Fellowship—a possible alternative to teaching. I've impressed them and have been offered a second interview. But on the drive home, I have a panic attack in the middle of the Leicester rush hour and spin the car around (2.6). I have a lucky escape but I quickly realise the attack is my unconscious telling me that I can't go through with the second interview, because I just can't believe in Biblical infallibility any more. It's a wake-up call about my shifting faith and when I see Sophie next, I explain it to her. She's glad I'm safe, but surprised by my confession.

"I never had you down for changing your mind about the Bible! But it means you're more like me now—a bit more liberal?"

"I suppose so, but I prefer the term 'neo-orthodox'; it sounds better. I guess I should start reading Karl Barth! The problem is, I don't know where it will all end—"

"In bed!" chirps Sophie. "It'll end up in bed! Let's move in together!"

*

Having both successfully completed our PGCE courses, Sophie is offered an RE post in a Grantham secondary school, whereas I accept a post at an independent school a few miles away with both teaching and chaplaincy work (2.6). The chapel has a broad-church Anglican tradition, so no one is too bothered about my private life. Just as well, for Sophie is forging ahead again and my head is in a spin once more. I accede to Sophie's suggestion and I move into her flat. We feel that we're a committed couple but as much as I long to have a sexual relationship, it's difficult to get rid of an evangelical conscience that's been troubling me for over a decade. So I suggest that I propose and that we get engaged, but without any plans to get married.

So that's our compromise. We get engaged, have a celebratory meal for two and then off to bed for real! For both of us, it's sheer relief and delight—made even more exciting for me, by feeling that I'm still breaking the rules! Sophie is absolutely kind, thoughtful and caring and can't do enough for me—almost too much! As for any questions that people might ask about a forthcoming marriage, we'll simply bat them into the long grass, although our close friends are made aware of our true situation—a never-ending engagement!

*

We have lots of fun, both in and out of bed. But after about a year, things start to change—on my side. I still see Sophie as lovely and as beautiful as ever, but my body doesn't desire her in the way it used to. Before long, it doesn't desire her at all. In response, Sophie tries even harder to tease and please me. But nothing seems to work for long and we're soon back at square one. We've simply no idea of what's wrong, or why, or what can be done. In the end, it becomes too embarrassing to talk about, so we start to detach ourselves from each other and begin to lead more separate lives. Sophie especially is devastated by my apparent rejection of her and her disappointment turns to criticism. After all, she still loves me and still wants to have sex with me, so who else is there to blame, apart from me? She's not quite so liberal now.

As for me, I have other pressing issues to think about, with dark clouds gathering on the horizon as my earlier trials of faith return to haunt me (2.6-9). Unlike for Sophie, *my* liberalising faith feels like the start of a slippery slope into agnosticism and beyond. Again, just like at Durham, I don't want to talk about it because to acknowledge my doubts will only make the problem seem all the more real. Neither do I want to undermine Sophie's contented faith by admitting to her my own increasing anxieties. So on this front too, we grow further apart and any real communication starts to dry up. Despite living together and being physically close to each other, as my faith declines so, it seems, does our relationship.

*

Eventually, I emerge from the agnosticism of *The Dark Night* (2.7), only to find myself in the angst of *The True Wilderness* (2.8), with my entire faith, identity and career about to be *Shipwrecked* (2.9). By now, Sophie and I are living different lives and sleeping in different beds. I find it difficult to live with the tension and my increasing inner loneliness. So I take up road-running, just to get out of the flat and be with myself. If I stay (like Sophie wants me to), it feels I am being buried alive. But if I leave, then what will become of me? How will I cope without my faith, my God or the church?

Two months later, I can't stand the tension and emptiness any more. So I move out of Sophie's flat and into a back-to-back terrace near the centre of Grantham. In the end, I'm keen to go—but oblivious of what's in store for me—in Desolation Row.

5. The Dating Game
Spring 1986

As she winds her window down, I speak my mind: "What time do you call this? You're twenty minutes late! I'm just about to leave!"

"You ignorant man! My son was sick, I shouldn't really have left him to meet *you*!"

With her words ringing in my ears, she winds the window back up and with a screech of tyres, she's off! This is my very first *Dateline* date—it lasted about two and a half seconds.

*

A week after moving into Desolation Row (as I call it), my friend Mike (2.9) suggests that I join *Dateline*; he realises—before me—that I'm going to be very isolated and that no one will come knocking on my front door, apart from him, unless I do something about it. I'm very reluctant to join a dating agency as it feels humiliating that I've sunk so low. I've never met women in this way before—never needed to. I must be desperate. I *am* desperate—for love, friendship, affection, sex and a partner to live with—the whole works! So I take Mike's advice, and the advantage of an introductory offer, and receive my first six *Dateline* names and telephone numbers through the post.

For my second date, I'm less anxious and less wound-up, and she arrives on time. Attractive, well-manicured and well-spoken, this date is much better and lasts almost forty minutes. But for much of the conversation, her eyes seem fixed on the barman, and although she's young and attractive, I've absolutely no interest in her.

Back home, I wonder why this is and arrive at some depressing conclusions. Firstly, I realise that I had nothing positive to say about myself: I'm an ex-football fan, an ex-Anglican minister, an ex-partner and an ex-teacher-chaplain. I'm an ex-parrot—I've ceased to be!

Secondly, it seems that there wasn't much wrong with her life—she was just lacking a fella.

Whereas my life is a total mess. We had nothing in common. I'm vulnerable and she's sorted. No wonder she was more interested in the barman, and why I was more interested in finishing my drink and going home. In future, I need to date women who are also vulnerable so that I can connect with them. I've learnt something. Nevertheless, back home, I feel empty, lonely and wretched. So I give *Dateline* a miss for a week. In any case, I've got a couple of teaching interviews to prepare for.

*

Several weeks later, my phone rings; it's a *Dateline* lady phoning me! Diana has the most eloquent, well-spoken yet empathetic voice; in fact, very similar to her namesake, the Princess of Wales. I'm entranced as we talk effortlessly for a whole hour, and then again the next day. We agree to meet the following Sunday in Nottingham. I wonder if she will look like the Princess of Wales? It's sort of possible because for my next *Dateline* contacts, I had asked to meet only those ladies who describe themselves as *very* attractive. If that's how they rate themselves, it's good enough for me and it does away with the need to fiddle about with photos, envelopes and stamps.

Upon arrival at the train station, I scan the platforms. A number of very attractive women, perhaps models, stride towards me, then stride past. An older woman in a bobble hat potters around, looking a bit disturbed as she struggles with a broken umbrella and a handbag that keeps falling open. I check the Arrivals board to see if Diana's train is late, but it's arrived on time. I see another slim and beautiful lady buying some flowers—she must be Diana. But just as I start to approach her, a tall and muscular guy turns up and lifts her off her feet! I don't think they're from *Dateline*!

By now, I'm somewhat perplexed and pace about, my anxiety increasing by the minute. The station has gone quiet. Then the woman in the bobble hat starts shuffling towards me and as she calls out my name, I suddenly realise…

Yes, it's Diana, but I cannot begin to match the dishevelled person in front of me with the Diana of the phone calls and my imagination. My heart sinks to my boots and I seriously contemplate doing a runner! But, distraught as I am with my 'date' (and my life), I cannot bring myself to do so. We walk around Nottingham for half an hour in the rain, call in at a dingy pub for a drink and say virtually nothing to each other. I just cannot get myself to engage with her on any level. I walk her back to the station and put her on the next train home. I apologise for the date and tell her that I'm in a bad way, which I know I am. I even think about returning to Sophie, but soon realise that's not a serious option. Going from one sort of emptiness to a lonelier sort of emptiness is no solution.

So much for the dating game on Desolation Row.

6. Love-Struck
July-December 1986

In a pub carpark on the outskirts of Nottingham, Francesca swings open the door of her red VW Golf. As she eases her way out, I can't help but notice the slit skirt and her long sensuous thigh. Perhaps she's meeting friends at a nightclub afterwards. She's as tall as me and with her natural blonde hair and good looks, she appears more like a model than a mental health nurse. Not that I really know what a mental health nurse is or does.

*

I'm back in the dating game after my earlier disappointments, thinking that at some point my luck will change. I contacted Francesca on a Friday, suggesting that we should exchange photos first, but she was keen to meet the next day. I'm very pleasantly surprised when I see her striking appearance, but I wonder if she's out of my league. She appears quite charming and we settle down to exchanging basic information over drinks. She's married, but her husband left her after a brief affair and is now in the Middle East as an oil engineer. She wanted children but he didn't, which was a problem. She doesn't expect to see him again and she's starting divorce proceedings—but I hope he doesn't suddenly turn up out of the blue! She does her mental health nursing in a local hospital, a job she really enjoys as it's so person-centred.

I tell her about my various 'ex' roles, but thankfully, I'm no longer an ex-teacher as I've recently had a successful interview at a large, local secondary school. So I'm an RE teacher again—not ideal for me, but it's all I can do so I'll just have to grin and bear it (5.1). Unlike my previous dates, Francesca seems genuinely interested in me and why my life has turned out the way it has. I'm not yet ready to talk about it, so I change the subject—but I appreciate her asking.

I'm starting to realise why she's a mental health nurse; I bet she's good at her job.

After a few drinks and feeling more relaxed, she suggests we carry on chatting at a nightclub, as she knows a few in Nottingham. I take this as a positive sign and go with the flow. I like her smile and the way she's looked at me a few times, and I try to match her moves on the dance floor. I'm half-expecting her to drift off with some handsome guy, but she seems pretty fixed on me and, as the evening wears on, we settle down on a sofa to chat. We think about calling it a night, but she cuddles up close, then kisses me on the lips. I reciprocate, overjoyed at how the date is turning out as I lap up her attention and affection.

"You're a special sort of guy, not like most men who come here. Can we meet again?" I walk her back to her car, high on hope, and wondering what the future may hold.

*

Our second date has to wait until ten days later, due to her shifts, and she comes over to my house; fortunately, it's dark so Desolation Row doesn't look quite so…desolate! The house has recently been redecorated, so the inside looks reasonably smart. As we settle down over coffee, she gives me one of her lovely warm smiles before asking me why I gave up the church. Now, for the first time, I feel I can talk to someone without any fear of judgement. With her gentle questioning and empathetic manner, I start to open up and pour out all the doubts and conflicts I've felt over the previous five years. It's truly liberating, as she starts to unlock my years in the religious and emotional wilderness. On several occasions, I'm close to tears as it's still very raw. I wonder what she'll think of me, but she reassures me with a hug and with those warm smiles and penetrating eyes. She's the first person that I can really trust and tell everything to—it's a truly amazing feeling!

After a natural break in the conversation, I go to the kitchen to replenish our cups and plates. When I return, she's rearranged herself on the sofa and invites me to snuggle down next to her.

"I think we've done enough talking for now, but we'll carry on next time. I've got something to show you, so budge over." She raises her slender legs in the air, allowing her slinky red dress to slip down to her waist. I'm shocked!

"You're not wearing any knickers!"

"Ha ha! I knew they'd be coming off, so why bother putting any on? But I've got some in my bag for the morning!" With that, she pulls me down and starts undressing me and before long, we're enjoying uninhibited sex on the floor. We hardly sleep a wink that night as we luxuriate in the warmth of our bodies while the loving continues until dawn starts to break.

*

The following week, we chat on the phone every day and express our love for each other. The next time we meet, it's at her place in Nottingham. It's a spacious town house, where she and her husband lived before he left. She greets me in her dressing gown, having just had a shower, following a long day at work. I wait downstairs while she changes.

"Jamie, shut your eyes. I'm coming down now—no peeping!" I sense her presence.

"Okay, stand up now and open your eyes!"

There in front of me is Francesca—in a shiny black catsuit with a full-length zip. Her sleek body is perfectly sculpted; she plays with the zip fastener underneath her chin, before she starts to slowly pull it down.

"I saw this in town at the weekend and thought you'd like it—what do you think?"

"It's amazing—I love it—what a body you have! The catsuit's nice as well!"

Francesca continues to slowly pull on the zip until both breasts are exposed. She pulls my head into her cleavage. "There you go, enjoy your meal. Breakfast is coming later!"

After my 'meal' is over, she continues to unzip herself past her navel and right down to her crotch, and again, no knickers. She unzips each leg, then, completely naked, takes me by the hand and leads me up the stairs.

It's a long, lazy, wonderful night. She's clearly far more experienced than me, although I'm keen to learn! Eventually, by spooning naked together, we get a few hours of sleep. In the morning, she brings me breakfast in bed, before continuing where we left off—until noon. Over lunch, she continues her gentle questioning about my loss of faith, loss of friends and the decline of my relationship with Sophie. Feeling that I can completely trust her and that she will listen and not condemn, I open up even more. But it's still scary, for this is something the like of which I've never experienced before.

"It's as though, as I was losing my faith, I was losing interest in Sophie too. I guess I didn't need Sophie like I needed God. That sounds crackers! But I just didn't have those loving feelings any more. Is that weird or what!" I also ask Francesca about her own marriage and her husband's affair, but she's less forthcoming about that, so I don't push it.

*

For the following months, we keep to similar arrangements: meeting once or twice a week, staying over with each other at weekends, while Francesca continues to gradually unlock my years of stress and pain. I'm utterly and overwhelmingly in love with her and nothing I've experienced in football, religion or previous relationships can begin to match the depths of my feelings or gratitude. For the first time in my life, I'm discovering intimacy, not primarily sexual intimacy (though that's nice too!) but personal intimacy, sharing my deepest thoughts and feelings and being accepted for who I am. I'm convinced I'm the happy beneficiary of Francesca being a mental health nurse—she certainly has something to work on with me!

Throughout these months, we also share our common interests in popular culture, mainly music and the occasional film. I'm starting to rebuild my 60s pop collection—the one that I gave away as a teenager—but adding 80s hits as well: Jennifer Rush, Kim Wilde, Erasure and the Pet Shop Boys.

I've found my soulmate at last and, I'm daring to hope, a partner for life. I don't need Jesus to save me, just Francesca. Jesus was confusing but Francesca is liberating—and real! I mention the possibility of a future together and perhaps moving in, but she doesn't take me up on it. I'm not too bothered as I'm as happy as a sand-boy and just love buying her flowers and enjoying her understanding and affection.

*

Then, on Christmas Eve, she arrives at my place to go out together, as it's a lovely sunny day. But I can tell that something is wrong—it's written all over her face and body. She sits down next to me and she's very emotional.

"Jamie, I love you to bits, but all this—it's too much for me—as I've not really recovered from my husband leaving. And now he wants to get back with me. He's apologised for his affair and says he's matured a lot in the Middle East. He wants to come back, settle down and have children.

"We'd been together for eight years, most of which were very happy. So I've got to give our marriage another chance. I'm truly very sorry."

I'm completely knocked sideways by this. I can hardly believe what I'm hearing—can hardly even breathe! Like other traumatic events in my life, I hadn't seen it coming.

"And what about me?" I plead, almost in tears.

"Jamie, you're a lovely, open and honest guy, and I've loved all of our time together. You'll find someone else, I know you will!"

We discuss the situation from every angle for over an hour. But I can see her mind is made up, so I'm only prolonging the agony. I watch in disbelief as she collects her things and throws them in her red VW Golf, before returning to me for a final hug and kiss. Then she's off, while I'm left shell-shocked and rooted to the spot. Too numb to feel the pain—that will come later. But what can I do? Where can I go?

I'm in Heartbreak Hotel on Desolation Row.

7. The Girl Next Door
Saturday, 3rd January 1987

"Hello, it's good to see you," Maggie greets me before leading me into her counselling room with its bright retro prints, potted plants and flowers. Maggie is younger than I was expecting—tall and slim, with a floral dress and large earrings—there's a decidedly hippie feel to the place.

I had struggled on for ten long days since Francesca's departure, feeling like one of the living dead—a zombie-like existence in a wasteland where all hope is lost—and at least as bad as my worst days in Durham. Francesca had been everything to me for the six months we had spent together, and now she's gone, and I'm nothing. Suicidal thoughts keep returning as I see no future without her. In the end, I break down and realise that my only hope is to see Maggie, a psychotherapist recommended by Mike's parents. I can't believe I've sunk so low—I need a miracle to save me on Desolation Row.

*

At the end of the first session, I ask Maggie whether I should continue with *Dateline*, and she advises against it, saying that I should learn to nurture myself and not be risking any further rejections. However, I've a yearning to have some feminine warmth in my life after Francesca's departure. One of my remaining *Dateline* contacts particularly intrigues me, as her address is literally around the corner from Heartbreak Hotel—my Grantham home. It would be nice to have a girlfriend so close! So I ignore Maggie's advice and make the phone call.

Marie answers, and she agrees it would be good to meet up as friends as we live so close. She's younger than me and is still at Nottingham University, having been away for a year for an archaeological dig and further study in Athens. She's now into her fourth year and most of her contemporaries have already graduated and have moved on. She seems appreciative of my friendship and we start going to the pub and to an occasional film together. I'm still hurting like hell about Francesca, but I keep it to myself as best I can. Marie, though petite and attractive, has nothing of the star-quality of Francesca, but I sense that she's out for some fun after a lonely time in Athens.

After arriving back at my house after our first night out, she starts coming on to me and I neither object nor resist. It's good to feel skin-to-skin contact again, although neither of us are in love, and the love-making can't compare with my times with Francesca. On another occasion, she takes me to her student room, which fulfils a fantasy of mine—to have sex in a student room on a university campus, which I'd never done before. All those wasted years of repressive religious restrictions! But the experience is far from a fantasy as I'm increasingly depressed over Francesca. The more I pretend to Marie, the more I miss Francesca. In the end, I admit that I've not gotten over Francesca, not by a mile, and that I'm going for weekly counselling. Marie is not really surprised and thereafter, backs away from me. However, she tells me that her cousin, Therese, needs a squash partner and running companion. Would I be interested?

I'm up for both, especially when I meet Therese for the first time. Although older than Marie, she's fresh-faced, very attractive and full of energy! We go road-running and play squash a couple of times and she puts a smile on my face, for the first time in a long while. She's very chatty and when I'm with her, I temporarily forget Francesca for an hour or so, which is a great relief. But when I try to get close to her, she pulls away and suddenly announces that she's met a new boyfriend at work, and that she's not able to see to see me anymore. Naturally, I'm upset all over again and my depression about Francesca seems darker and deeper than ever. I seem to have no inner resources to save me from my brief, exhilarating highs and sudden catastrophic lows and I can see why Maggie advised me to discontinue my *Dateline* activities. I do just that, despite increasing the risk of loneliness and further obsessive thinking about Francesca.

It's now the end of the month and a normal Saturday routine for me: my weekly session with Maggie in the morning, followed by my weekly shop and an afternoon of TV sport. It's the FA Cup and suddenly, one scoreline on the BBC vidiprinter catches my eye and gives me a jolt:

Manchester United 0 Coventry City 1

It's a shock result, and suddenly there's a lump in my throat and a tear in my eye (4.3).

8. Uproar

Several Years Later

"Put Sam back!"
"Pardon?"
"You heard. Put Sam [the cat] back on the bed. He was there before you!"
I'm at a loss what to say or how to respond.

*

With the start of the new decade, I move out of Desolation Row and into a better part of town where I feel more at home. I join a Nottingham Singles group, although it's not really my scene, as I struggle with small talk with complete strangers. But at one of their evenings, I meet Millie, who's very friendly. She's a bright and bubbly lady, chic and attractive and a solicitor of Afro-Caribbean heritage. She's the centre of much male attention so I'm happily surprised that, after a couple of weeks, she's latched on to me as her friend and confidante. Before the month is out, we are also lovers, and for me there's no turning back. I'm hooked! We arrange to go on a weekend break together and that's when I get the first inkling of trouble. On the very day we make the booking, I'm faced with the 'cat on the bed' incident—and I'm at a loss about what to do or how to respond.

I've not seen Millie as assertive as this before. She's usually fun, light-hearted and positive, both in and out of the bedroom. I'm sure I'd moved Sam off the bed before—so what's got into her? I resign myself to a night on the floor, but when Sam meows to be let out, our normal sleeping arrangements are resumed. But I don't sleep well. This is not the first time that Millie's been a bit 'odd' with me; the previous week, she came out with "all football fans are morons", knowing full well that I'm a keen Coventry City supporter—it's like a red rag to a bull!

Perhaps I should respond in kind, but I don't want our blossoming romance to descend into insults and arguments, and all out of nothing. Eventually, I go to see Maggie to see if she can shed any light on the situation.

"From what you say, it sounds like a variant of *Uproar*—when someone feels threatened by a partner getting too close, they throw a spanner in the works, so as to keep some distance in the relationship. Of course, it's all done at an unconscious level; you can read about it in Eric Berne's *Games People Play* [56]. And if you get the opportunity, you could ask Millie about her childhood—it may have been quite difficult."

"Like mine, you mean?"

"Possibly like yours, but it's hard to say, given her very different background."

It's on the weekend holiday itself when an opportunity to talk to her presents itself.

*

It's wonderful to be alone with Millie for a whole weekend, without any distractions, and I tease her about the limitless opportunities we have for sex—but the lady is not for teasing.

"Sex is for night-time, and even then, only if you're lucky! Daytime is for walking!"

Again, I'm shocked. Back home, the time of day and location had never stopped us—apart from the cat on the bed. Sex was fun, flirty and adventurous—until now. The weekend didn't get any better and by the end of it, I felt so demoralised by her random criticisms that I decided to end our relationship there and then—and we drove back home in silence. What we had enjoyed for the first few months had now disappeared. The weekend away had clearly been a bad idea.

Back home, we both lie low for a few days before making contact. Millie comes around to my place and we talk. I listen as empathetically as I can, realising that there may be a story behind Millie's behaviour. There is. A story of well-meaning parents (like mine) but whom Millie felt never really loved her unconditionally. She always had to put on a little-girl performance to attract attention and win parental approval: to dress prettily, be 'sugar and spice and all things nice', to sing and dance—it was exhausting. She felt she had never been valued just for being herself.

She finished her story, close to tears, and thanked me for listening; she had never told this to anyone before. She apologised for her behaviour on the holiday, caused by her not daring to get too close to me. Yes, she liked sex, of course, but found it easier when it was more of a performance than an emotional encounter. That's why she kept pushing me away—too far away it seems, as she hadn't intended us to split up.

"So can we restart our relationship?" she asks.

We get back together immediately and things seem better than ever. We communicate more deeply, Millie sparkles again and tells me more about her childhood. And there's no more *Uproar*! Perhaps now, this relationship might develop into the long-term relationship that I had hoped for with Francesca. But I couldn't have been more wrong.

*

After a few blissful months, Millie is struggling again and decides that she wants me to be a close and long-term friend, but no longer a sexual partner. I'm deeply hurt, but decide to 'hang in there', hoping that this is just another developmental milestone for Millie that will be dealt with in due course. I don't want to abandon her just because of the lack of sex. Moreover, after all our conversations together, I am now starting to build up an interesting psychological portrait of her—though it's far from complete. One thing I want to know is what attracts her to certain men—her ex-husband, for example—and also me?

"At university, he was a loner—stuck in his books all day and he never went out. I felt sorry for him and thought I could help him."

And what about me?

"You seemed lonely too—finding it difficult to talk to anyone in the Singles group. I thought you needed warming up." I detect a pattern emerging; Millie is a charitable soul and is always helping good causes: women's groups, ethnic minority groups and the like—the sort of work that I could never imagine myself doing. It's very impressive, but I'm starting to connect a few dots: her childhood, charity work and attraction to lonely, needy people.

In the New Year, Millie comes to me with a confession—that she has recently met someone else who is in dire straits. He's a virtual recluse, with no job, no social life and heavily reliant on drink to keep himself going. He's recently attempted suicide. Millie admits that she's fallen for him, even though her advances aren't reciprocated. She wants to help him, to change him and bring him in from the cold. I can tell that her new friendship has impacted negatively upon us. I suggest to Millie that she has 'normalised me' and that, having helped me feel more positive about myself, I had stopped being as attractive to her. Reluctantly, she agrees: "But that's just the way I am—I can't help it!"

Finally, Millie breaks up with me, although we continue to meet and talk as friends—but that's all. I keep hanging in there and hoping for the best—but nothing changes.

*

For a while, I'm disconsolate about Millie; I had entertained such high hopes! However, my disappointment is offset to a certain extent by my interest in her psychological history and make-up. I start to make a list of key issues, when a bell rings in my head: I've seen this type of list before, but where? I rack my brain until I have it: *Women Who Love Too Much* by Robin Norwood [57].

Someone had lent it to me once. So I'm quickly along to *Borders* bookshop and, back home, I scour the first chapter, in which I find a list of fifteen psychological characteristics of women who try to make up for their lack of love in childhood by helping others, especially needy men, in order to boost their own self-esteem. At a quick glance, I identify twelve of these features in Millie—and a few in myself, apart from the charity and helping elements, that is! I read the whole book in a few days, seeing it as a reflection of Millie's relationships with her various men-friends, including me.

*

At about the same time, a sensational new book arrives in the public arena that stuns the nation: *Diana: Her True Story* [58]. I'm fascinated by Princess Diana's personal journey: the rejection by her parents, her search for self-esteem through her charitable works and her falling head over heels in love with an emotionally unavailable man, Prince Charles. Despite their very different backgrounds, it's a similar story to Millie's, and to the many accounts contained in *Women Who Love Too Much*. Therefore, in meeting Millie, I didn't just meet a strange lady I couldn't understand, but I'd fallen for someone who had suffered emotional deprivation in childhood leading to problems in adulthood like others—including the most recent addition to the Royal Family!

Given my greater understanding, I start to write up Millie's life-story as an informal psychological case-study, which I simply entitle *Uproar*. I go into some detail about the picture that has emerged from our many conversations and I eventually present it to Millie. There's a few details I've misunderstood but overall, she agrees that I've given a fair picture of her life-story and how her childhood has affected her as an adult. Whether she can do anything about it, even if she wants to, is another matter however. But she thanks me for the understanding and insight.

I feel that I've learnt a lot being with Millie. And I'm about to learn a good deal more, as I decide to join a local dating agency, where I soon meet Karla and enter into another engaging, yet unconventional, relationship—and where, thankfully, there's no *Uproar* at all!

9. Surprise! Surprise!

1992–3

Karla's jet-black curls are unmistakable, along with her tight leather skirt and jacket, as she strides towards me outside All Saints Church in Huntingdon town centre—our agreed rendezvous. She greets me with kisses on both cheeks, hooks up my arm and whisks me off to her favourite café.

*

"So Jamie, how many one-night stands have you had?"

This is NOT the standard first question on a normal first date! I'm surprised, shocked even, yet I'm secretly delighted at Karla's free spirit—and intrigued. After giving my answer of nil, I return the question across the table:

"Me? Oh, hundreds! You see, I studied maths at Cambridge a decade ago, and I was outnumbered by 10:1 men to women. And I love men! So I had a great time and always had a man, or two, on the go. But they didn't last long. I wanted to suck *all* the sweets in the sweet shop, so to speak!"

I'm immediately into Karla. The problem is that I'm still in love with Millie, as we are continuing to meet up, and I cling to the hope that she might come back. Karla quickly picks up on this and seems sympathetic, while I worry that I might have already ruined the date. But apparently not.

At the end of the evening, as we are chatting in her car, I get my second surprise when she tells me about the lingerie she bought earlier in the day.

"Would you like to see it?" she asks. I would—expecting her to open up her shopping bags.

"Close your eyes then." I sense some shuffling going on and something being dropped onto the seat behind. When I open my eyes, behold her lingerie! In flamingo pink and white lace stockings and suspenders, very brief knickers and matching bra, with her dress on the back seat, obviously.

She tells me that I can touch as well as look but, taken aback by her invitation, I think the better of it; there's plenty to look at, as it is!

*

I've met up with Karla through a Midlands dating agency—not *Dateline*—which means I get a lot more information as well as contact details. Her self-description includes the fact that she is a single mum with two young children, as well as being outgoing, music-loving, very attractive and intelligent. Her reply to my initial letter came handwritten and on flowery, perfumed notepaper. The accompanying photo suggested that she was indeed stunningly attractive—and I like the line where she admits she can't find men 'on my wavelength' in nightclubs—perhaps not surprising for a Cambridge maths graduate. I hope that *I'm* on her wavelength! But there's a problem. Two, in fact.

After I have inspected and approved of her lingerie, I ask her for another date. Naturally. But for her, the hour's drive between our homes in Grantham and Huntingdon is a problem. She doesn't want to introduce another boyfriend to her young sons and the financial cost (of petrol and childminding) of her coming to Grantham on a regular basis would be too great, as she only works part-time. The other problem is that she is still in touch with her ex-husband and hopes one day to get back with him, although that is unlikely in the foreseeable future. Therefore, she doesn't see a long-term future for us. I strongly suspect that I'm being fobbed off as she knew where I lived from the outset. She's just not interested in me. I put this to her and she protests strongly; indeed, she has seemed very positive towards me throughout the three hours of our date. I return home disappointed and confused, intrigued by such a different and slightly crazy lady. But then, I'm a slightly crazy man.

The next day I have an idea, which I put to her over the phone. It will test her motives as well.

"If you come to see me, I'll pay your expenses—childminding, petrol, whatever. How about coming over once a month for a few hours? What do you think?" She calls me back and thinks it's a good idea. She will come up to Grantham on the first Sunday of each month, 7 to 10 pm. As she's doing all the driving, I'm happy enough to cover her expenses. Perhaps she likes me after all.

*

135

On the first Sunday, she arrives right on time at my terraced town house, which is a big improvement on Desolation Row! As she peels off her coat, I'm in for another surprise—a bright pink dress, extremely short, with a plunging neckline. She's hot! And I'm feeling pretty hot too!

"And guess what lingerie I'm wearing? But that's for later."

We order a Chinese take-away and settle down to eat and chat. We've a lot to talk about. After an hour or so, she announces: "Well, Jamie, that's enough talking for one night—where's the bedroom?"

So off we go, hand-in-hand, up the stairs, to undress each other and get down to bodily delights. We're right in the middle of love-making when something happens and I suddenly withdraw and sit up.

"I can't do it! I can't do it! I'm still in love with Millie!"

We put some dressing gowns on as we chat and I realise that I've completely messed up, and that our first Sunday date will probably be our last. I'm expecting Karla to rush off but she doesn't.

"Jamie, I knew you were still in love with Millie so I was half-expecting that to happen. It's happened to lots of men that I've been with and to me as well on occasions. So, unless you *want* me to go, I'll stay, if that's all right." I can hardly believe my ears! Such wisdom! Such generosity—while I'm thinking that all is lost. I'm most appreciative of her attitude and support and tell her so.

We continue to meet every first Sunday of the month, with the same familiar pattern, although occasionally we go to a show in Nottingham. Our talk is wide-ranging about schools, society, psychology and literature. Her sexuality is wide-ranging too, from her dress sense (hot pants to exotic lingerie) to her bedroom experience—of which I'm a keen student. Thoughts of Millie start to fade and occasionally, I find myself developing feelings for Karla and give her a broad hint to test her reaction. But her reply is always the same—a gentle reminder that she hopes to get back with her husband, especially for her boys' sakes. That's okay. I'm glad of the reminder not to fall in love with her and that sex can still be enjoyable, even passionate, without the need for emotional entanglements. I really enjoy the warm friendship and good sex, without being on an emotional rollercoaster. I'm learning a lot and my traditional attitudes to love, relationships and sex are being transformed.

*

In the New Year, other events trigger a cathartic experience for me (4.7) and I start to write stories about my passionate life so far. Karla takes away copies of my latest efforts and reads them at home. The following month, she discusses aspects of them with me and occasionally suggests some improvements. It's clear she's read every word and she's very supportive about what I'm doing. I'm very grateful and appreciate her wisdom. At the other end of the literary scale, in the summer she sends me a holiday postcard showing some beautiful bikini-clad bottoms on a beach. Her message is simple: *Wish you were here—but we'll 'come' together soon! Love Karla xxx.*

As autumn drifts into winter, we agree that we will go our separate ways after Christmas, for Karla is hoping for a Christmas reconciliation with her husband. But there are still a couple of surprises for me before we part. The first of these is my reading of *John Bowlby & Attachment Theory*, which has recently been published [59]. It confirms in great detail the direction of my thinking since meeting Millie. It's the most influential book I've ever read and it has a huge impact on my life (4.9). I share all of this with Karla at our last meeting, just before Christmas.

The second surprise is with myself. As we say our final goodbyes, I'm not distraught or devastated by losing Karla as was typical of previous relationships. Rather, I'm calm, collected and accepting of the situation. I'm extremely grateful to Karla for her openness, honesty and support over the past eighteen months, but I feel ready now to stand on my own two feet. I've experienced a very unconventional relationship but, in many respects, it's the best I've had. As we kiss goodbye for the last time, there are no regrets. With Attachment Theory to delve into, it's time to try to make sense of my crazy, passionate life.

*

However, never in my wildest dreams did I think that, in less than three years' time, I would actually be *teaching* Attachment Theory for 'A' level, as the head of a new psychology department in my school (5.4).

The surprises keep on coming.

10. Romantic Passions: Review

* If you are thinking of taking 'The Love Quiz' (Appendix A), this would be the best point at which to do this, before reading on.

A. Romance and Attachment Theory: Basic Principles

i.   John Bowlby always believed that basic attachments in infancy would affect the rest of a person's life. Since the mid-1980s, a great deal of research has been undertaken on this matter, especially in respect of adult romantic relationships. This research has shown Bowlby to be right. In most books today about love and romance, there will usually be a section devoted to Attachment Theory, often starting with 'The Love Quiz' of Hazan and Shaver (1987) that yielded such interesting results. Three important principles from Attachment Theory are relevant here: *the Attachment hierarchy; Romantic attachment styles*; and *'Earned' secure attachment.* These basic principles will be explained and then applied to the specific relationships described in Chapter 3.

It should be noted, however, that recent attachment research reveals adult attachments to be more malleable and fluid than childhood attachments [60]. The main reasons for this are the increased number of potential attachment figures and the more reflective nature of adulthood, which allows for the selection of attachment figures for specific needs. Even so, for the majority of adults, a spouse or romantic partner is the most commonly preferred attachment figure.

ii.   Bowlby proposed that an **Attachment hierarchy** exists for all children. Thus, although a child may have a number of attachment figures in his or her life, there was always *one* that was preferred, the loss of whom would cause a great deal of distress, even despair. Bowlby called this preference for one attachment figure *monotropy* and the preferred figure—*the principal attachment figure.* Usually, this would be the child's mother or father. Others, such as the other parent, other relatives or childminders may be *subsidiary attachment figures* [61]. For Bowlby himself, his nanny, Minnie, was his principal attachment figure for the first four years of his life, with his parents (less loving and less available) being subsidiary figures [62]. Such a hierarchy also exists for adults, but it may be more changeable and flexible than for children, for the reasons given in *i* (b) above.

iii. **Romantic attachment styles**: In the mid-1980s, American attachment researchers, Hazan and Shaver, used the infant attachment types of Mary Ainsworth [63], to discover whether these continued into adulthood, in particular into adult romantic relationships. They found a strong correlation between infant and adult attachments, and subsequent research has supported their findings. Three corresponding attachment styles have been identified, and the research has indicated that a child's attachment type in infancy is likely to lead to a corresponding romantic style in adulthood [64]. These three romantic styles can be summarised as follows:

- *Securely attached*: People have healthy balance between wanting closeness and being comfortable with independence. If a relationship ends, there is some distress but not despair.
- *Avoidantly attached:* People avoid closeness and are excessively independent. Feelings are difficult to acknowledge or process. Relationship endings are met with indifference.
- *Anxiously (ambivalently) attached:* People are insecure and clingy and may want to 'merge' with their partner, so as not to lose them. They seek dependency, not independence. Endings may be traumatic and may lead to despair.

The particular combination of romantic attachment styles within a relationship may provide clues to that relationship's trajectory—towards longevity or towards breakdown.

iv.   **'Earned' secure attachment** is a relatively recent arrival in attachment discourse. Evidence has been gathered about individuals with insecure attachments in childhood who nevertheless 'do well' and become securely attached in adulthood. Reasons for this include a settled relationship to a securely attached partner [65] or the achievement of *autobiographical competence* by coming to a mature and balanced view of one's life, with the ability to process emotionally painful events [66].

B. Romance and Attachment Theory Applied (3.1–3.9)

i.   By the time I met Celia, my principal attachment was to evangelical religion, God and Jesus Christ. I was unquestioning about my conversion process, with Jesus Christ becoming my 'sure foundation' and 'cornerstone'. Through religion, I had *earned* a 'secure base', which enabled me to do my early evangelistic work (2.3). Celia was an important, yet subsidiary attachment figure, and would remain so. Everything about Celia suggests that she was also securely attached, so our secure-secure attachments facilitated a happy early relationship for over eighteen months. However, the Sargant lecture in Durham (2.4) demolished my earned security in one go, so I reverted to my more familiar anxious-ambivalent attachment type. Celia remained a subsidiary attachment figure and was, unwittingly, a 'safe haven' throughout my difficulties of faith. But we were no longer on the same attachment page and this, I believe, is the underlying reason why she 'fell out of love' with me. The pain of her departure was eased by my renewed attachment to my principal attachment figure; namely, evangelical religion in the form of God and Jesus Christ (2.5).

ii.   With girlfriend Holly and long-term fiancée Sophie, evangelical religion continued to be my principle attachment object, and again they became subsidiary attachment figures. With both, in the initial stages, there was a shared and enjoyable sensuality, probably made more intense because of the pre-marital sex prohibition, which was adhered to—at least in terms of full intercourse. But in both, passion died down. With Holly, this was probably due to a lack of personal connection in the first place, which was exemplified and aggravated by her decision to move to

Newcastle, as well as the widening political gap. This was easy enough to understand at the time.

iii.   With Sophie, however, the lessening and eventual loss of desire on my part was completely unexpected and confusing—and neither of us had any insight into the issue [67]. With hindsight, it seems that there were a number of forces at work: 1. Sophie's over-availability, especially in the bedroom, was counter-productive. For reasons concerning my mother's *un*availability in infancy (1.1) I had no neural network that could respond to Sophie's unconditional acceptance of me (see also 5.7 and 7.10). 2. My ever-darkening storm clouds of religious doubt led to my being depressed—due to the threat of me losing my principle attachment figure. All my passion was spent on trying to save my faith and religious vocation—and not on Sophie. 3. In trying to spare Sophie the same crisis of faith, I cut myself off from her—as I had done with Celia previously for the same reason. 4. The resulting distance between us led Sophie into a 'critical parent' role, as I increasingly felt more like a little boy. 5. In the larger analysis, my relationship with Sophie failed when my principal attachment failed; i.e., my attachment to 'God'. It had been evangelical religion that had kept me motivated throughout our time together, and when that failed, our relationship failed. Our relationship had, in fact, been dependent upon my religious attachment for its energy. So in losing one, I lost them both.

iv.   I arrived in the aptly nicknamed Desolation Row, truly desolate. For the first time in a quarter of a century—since I had started (then stopped) supporting Coventry City—I had no principal attachment figure. I was floating on a featureless sea without a ship in sight, let alone a lifeboat, and drowning was an ever-present possibility. I had virtually no subsidiary attachments either. My parents were still alive and well, but they were the last people I would talk to. Mike was supportive and suggested I join *Dateline*, but within a few months he'd moved to London and contact thereafter was rare. Curly, my long-standing friend, and his wife, Joanna, were at the end of a telephone, but were having their own problems.

I started the dating game (3.5) with the aim of finding my partner for life. There was a God-shaped hole in my life (a rather large hole) and it needing filling. I was desperate not to be alone—desperate for a personal principal attachment figure. I soon discovered (on my second date) that I needed a vulnerable, insecure partner—like me—with whom I had something in common. I entered into the realm of fantasy about Diana, and was bitterly disappointed, both with my date and with myself, as despair continued to haunt me. Until, that is, I met Francesca.

v.   Francesca immediately became my principal attachment figure and, it would seem, the only 'flesh and blood' human being ever to become so. For, unlike Celia and Sophie, she arrived *after* my institutional attachment to religion was over, but *before* those future institutional attachments that would dominate the rest of my life. In this sense, Francesca was unique. In retrospect, it would seem that she was securely attached, with a strong 'nurturing parent' within—well equipped to care for my needy 'inner child', as her role in mental healthcare also suggested. However, she had recently suffered from her husband's affair and departure so she had her own vulnerabilities, which gave us both experiences of loss. Her wacky free spirit reminded me of mine: of my teenage passion for Coventry City and of my enthusiastic days as 'God's Evangelist'. We *seemed* a perfect match!

vi.   Moreover, the plentiful sex reassured me (after a sexually problematic time with Sophie) that I could function quite normally, and the skin-to-skin body contact was hugely nurturing for me, having lived the previous decade mostly in my head. In short, she quickly replaced 'God', church and faith as my attachment figures—so I was desperate to cling onto her and hoped we would become life-long partners. But that, it seems, was the problem. Who could possibly bear the weight of those roles and my expectations? In any case, we were *not* perfectly matched after all, for the relationship was very skewed—with her (nurturing) 'parent' caring for my (needy) 'child'—not adult to adult. Francesca brought a great deal to the relationship, whereas I brought little, mainly my neediness.

In the end, being my principal attachment figure became too much for her. I only have her word about 'the returning husband' story. It's possible that she just wanted out and the husband story was the kindest way to let me down. Whichever way it was, I bore her no ill-will as she had given me all of herself for six months and had opened my eyes to a new world of intimacy, fun and love.

The crash, when it came, was soul-destroying. Indeed, it was the darkest of my dark days—with sleepless nights and many, long, depressing days to get through. When I was in Durham, I still had Celia when I had 'lost' God, and by the time I lost Celia, I had found God again. But now, I had no God and no Francesca—a double loss, as I suffered separation-anxiety from two recent and hugely important attachment figures. And, lacking in self-esteem, I was dead-beat at the dead end of a dead-end street. My only hope was to see Maggie—in case she could help (4.1).

vii.   In meeting Marie, the girl next door, and her cousin, Therese, I went against Maggie's advice. But I had accepted that Marie would only be, at best, a friend (a subsidiary attachment figure) and that's how it was, despite becoming lovers for a short while. Francesca remained my principal attachment figure, even though she had left me. Things only started to change when I saw that Coventry City had beaten Manchester United in the F. A. Cup—and I sensed a stirring in the breeze, as patches of sky blue started to appear from behind the heavy rain-clouds of my life (4.3).

viii.   By the time I met Millie, I had re-attached to my beloved Coventry City, which became my principal institutional attachment once again (4.3). But the football club was still very poor at providing a meaningful social life for me, so a girlfriend/partner for life was still an urgent need.

ix.   Meeting Millie was a great joy—probably because of our common vulnerabilities in terms of past relationships. From the outset, it felt like an evenly balanced adult-to-adult relationship (or maybe child-to-child!) but her *Uproars* gave me cause for concern. For she could switch from the amorous and caring to the arrogant and critical at the drop of a hat—or a cat!

From an attachment perspective, she seemed ambivalently attached in the true meaning of the term, being 'strong in two directions', and in

143

quick succession! For me, it was like walking on eggshells. If Maggie was right about *Uproar* signalling a fear of intimacy, then it is not surprising that Millie unwittingly sabotaged our weekend away from the start, replete as it was with potential for romance and intimacy. Despite this setback, I grew in self-esteem as a result of being physically and psychologically close to her, whereas her self-esteem came from helping and hopefully changing an another unpromising, needy and avoidant man. We were two needy 'ambivalents', but wanting almost opposite things. I brought some understanding to her situation, which she appreciated, and our love-making was warm and tender, flooding my brain with oxytocin, the 'love hormone', which kept me nurtured, bonded and attracted to her. Unfortunately, this very closeness rendered me less attractive in her eyes, so off she went in search of a more damaged soul to save [68].

Another positive aspect of our nine-month relationship was Millie's openness to discussions about her childhood and the psychological legacy this had bequeathed her. It meant that we continued to talk well after our love affair was over and in this respect, she opened the door for me into understanding something about childhood development. On this basis, I wrote my case-study about her—and Princess Diana—which led me, eighteen months later, to Attachment Theory. It had been exactly the sort of relationship one should expect when two ambivalents get together! [69]

x.   I met Karla soon after Millie had broken up with me and it quickly became clear that any future relationship would be quite different from my recent experiences. Coventry City would remain my principal attachment figure and Karla would become an important and interesting subsidiary figure. Karla seemed secure in herself and knew her own mind. She provided a safe haven for me while I was still struggling over the loss of Millie. She also showed empathy where that was needed, and was positive and supportive about my cathartic, autobiographical stories (4.7). Her boundary lines about my 'not falling in love' with her constrained my neediness and she helped me enjoy the present rather than trying to predict and control the future. She got me thinking more clearly, and more open-mindedly, about friendship, sex and

144

relationships: there was now a new and exciting menu of relationship types to dine out on, rather than just reheating the same conventional meal—which, in my case, had only made me feel sick—love sick. [70] As a consequence of my unconventional eighteen months with Karla, I was feeling much better about myself. I had started on the long and winding road towards *earning* for myself a more secure attachment.

Summary:

1. My principal attachments throughout these years (1967-93) were to Coventry City F. C. and to evangelical religion, i.e., to institutions rather than to flesh and blood individuals.

2. My girlfriends were all subsidiary attachment figures (with one exception), although there was considerable variety in these relationships. Such variation is consistent with the more malleable and fluid nature of adult attachments as explained in i (b) above.

3. The exception was Francesca who, coming in between two institutional attachments, bore the full weight of being, for a while, my *only* attachment figure.

4. Therefore, the loss of Francesca was catastrophic, similar to my loss of faith at Durham.

5. Although remaining fundamentally anxiously/ambivalently attached myself, my relationships included women of all attachment types: secure, avoidant and ambivalent.

6. My later relationships with Millie and Karla helped me understand myself better; helped me think more maturely; and furthered my interest in developmental and life-course psychology.

7. Issues concerning my variable sexual responses seemed rather confusing and contradictory and they would return to haunt me later (5.6 and 7.7).

*

To support positive mental health:

Romantic and sexual relationships can enhance self-esteem. But be aware of becoming too dependent and/or clingy—for sudden loss (being dumped) may be overwhelming and lead to self-harm or even suicidal thoughts. Ideally, one needs to develop an inner core that is contented in itself and is happy either in or out of a romantic relationship. For those who are securely attached, this sense of self is already in place. For those insecurely attached, the need for love seems greater but with it, there is a greater vulnerability to rejection.

Beauty is not the basis for a long-lasting relationship—the nature and quality of that relationship is. All relationships change over time—some for the better, some for the worse. Working out what's changing and why is the tricky bit. And remember, there's never just *one* relationship—there's the relationship *as I see it* and the relationship *as my partner sees it*—and they may be surprisingly different from each other. Sharing these different perspectives is essential for the mental health of both partners, but such honest talking can often be difficult. Sometimes a therapist will be needed to help sort out what's going on and what can be done about it.

It must also be said that having a conventional relationship or marriage is no guarantee of its success, and unconventional relationships may work better for some people, including being single. A further alternative is becoming attached to an institution, of which there are myriads of possibilities—politics, religion and sport being just three popular examples. These may also provide meaningful friendships or help buffer the loss of a personal romance.

Chapter 4 ~ Therapies
1986–95

1. Psychotherapy

"James, I think you will find that if you want to move forwards, you will first have to look backwards."

Those are the words I remember most from my first therapy session some three decades ago—but they were the last words I wanted to hear. I wanted to be rescued from my agony now. I wanted a quick fix.

*

I arrive at Maggie's door in desperation, ten long days after Francesca had left me (3.7). I'm struggling to hold myself together and I doubt whether Maggie, with her hippie look, will be on my wavelength at all. She invites me to explain my situation, then bears the bad news:

"Jamie, it sounds to me that we're dealing with a bereavement, a profound and significant loss for you, and you don't know what to do."

I feel reassured that she's taking my situation seriously but am unprepared for what is to follow.

"Jamie, tell me something about your mother—what's she like?"

I can hardly believe my ears! I become very animated and angry and think about walking out.

"What a ridiculous question! My mother has nothing to do with my life and doesn't understand the first thing about me! So please move on and help me *now*!"

"James, I think you will find that if you want to move forwards, you will first have to look backwards—but we can leave this for now and return to it in a later session."

*

I see Maggie for an hour every Saturday morning for six months. Thereafter, every fortnight. She steers well clear of discussing my mother for several sessions, focussing more on my current isolation. I'm often in tears at the sheer loneliness I'm feeling. I want her to put an arm around me and give me a hug, but she remains stoically seated across from me and waits until I've regained some composure. These are dark, difficult sessions; although I always drive home with a new thought about to explode in my head, like a hand-grenade with the pin pulled. This keeps me coming back and however tough these sessions are, it's still the best hour of my week, given the discipline problems I'm having at my new school (5.1).

Eventually, she returns to the subject of my mother, by which time I have reassessed and think that there might be something in it. I've also had the time and mental space to recall my mother's oft-told story of her 'unforgettable night' (1.1). Maggie listens intently before speaking:

"It seems to me that just as you were starting to form some emotional bonds with your mother, these got seriously disrupted by her own traumatic experience and perhaps she was never able to connect with you properly after that. It sounds as though she was clinically depressed."

I can sense that Maggie thinks this to be important, but I don't see the link to my current situation and I remain hostile to all further questions about my mother.

*

I realise that my sessions with Maggie are essential for my well-being—for I have someone to talk to on a regular basis and she's making me think. But I'm disappointed that after a couple of months, I really don't feel much better—and I'm still obsessing about Francesca.

One thing in particular that intrigues me is Maggie's language. There are two terms she often uses that fascinate me, even though I don't understand them: 'free child' and 'critical parent'.

"Maggie, what do you mean by 'free child' and 'critical parent'?"

"Oh, they are terms from *Transactional Analysis*. Would you like a session on that? It might be useful." I would, and so we do (4.2).

*

Thereafter, my sessions with Maggie become brighter and more engaging. Much to the annoyance of my few friends and school colleagues, I start to quote Maggie on anything and everything to do with personal relationships—as she's become my new infallible Bible. But the star that is shining most brightly in the early days of my therapeutic journey is the guiding light of *Transactional Analysis*.

2. Transactional Analysis

* If you are thinking of taking the 'Ego-gram' exercise (Appendix B), this would be the best point at which to do this, before reading on.

"Hell's bells! It's obvious from this why you should never have been a minister!"

Maggie is studying the Ego-gram that I've just completed in pencil in under five minutes. I'm intrigued to know how she arrived at that conclusion so quickly. She shows me my Ego-gram.

"Just look at your Free Child—it's almost off the page! And your Critical Parent—you barely have one!"

"So what?" I ask. "I don't get it."

Maggie explains, "A minister is meant to be telling his congregation how to live a good Christian life by keeping to the straight and narrow—that's his Critical Parent at work. So your weak Critical Parent may partly explain your discipline problems at school. Whereas your strong Free Child would have encouraged your free thinking and break from the church."

*

Step by step, Maggie explains Eric Berne's post-Freudian model of human personality [71].

Within every human being, there are three inner selves: the *Parent* (nurturing and critical); the *Adult* (rational and information processing) and the *Child* (adaptive and free).

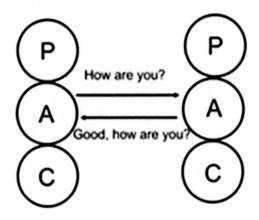

Diag. 1

Maggie then gets a piece of paper and draws circles and arrows to show how transactions emanate from one of these 'selves' and are directed towards a particular 'self' in the other person. Diagram 1 shows a simple *Adult to Adult* transaction, which is an example of a parallel transaction. Parallel transactions allow the dialogue to continue without difficulty, but crossed transactions cause problems, as in Diagram 2 below:

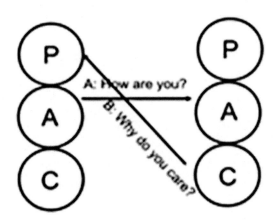

Diag. 2

Those who are well adjusted are able to move in and out of their various inner selves as appropriate and with ease. Less well-adjusted individuals tend to get stuck in one predominant role; for example, an overly caring person (strong Nurturing Parent) may get taken advantage of; a highly critical person (strong Critical Parent) may blame others without thinking first; or a fun-loving person who behaves impulsively (strong Free Child) may do so without thinking of the consequences of their actions. Thankfully, Maggie tells me that my rational, thinking Adult is very high and that, in the absence of a strong Critical Parent, it would limit the risks that my strong Free Child might undertake.

With this fairly basic understanding of T. A., I start to realise that my later problems with Sophie were to do with her Critical Parent talking down to my Child, and similarly with the church; as Maggie had already suggested, I was too free-spirited and too free-thinking for it to contain me within its bounds. My relationships with my parents told a similar story for I cannot recall any Adult to Adult conversation between us. It was always their Critical Parent talking down to my Child. No wonder that I've never felt grown up! It was to escape such transactional tyranny that I became a passionate football supporter at Coventry City, where my Free Child could live and breathe and have its being.

Maggie can see that I'm finding T. A. both interesting and illuminating. At last, a few things are starting to make sense. So she invites me to a Saturday morning T. A. conference for students and trainee psychotherapists—and I readily accept. On the day itself, I give her a hint that I might be in Free Child mode, as the night before I'd been at Highfield Road, Coventry, for the first time in thirteen years, roaring on my beloved Sky Blues towards F. A. Cup glory!

3. Coming Around Again
Carly Simon [72]
Highfield Road, Coventry,
Friday March 20, 1987

As the Sky Blues emerge from the players' tunnel and onto the pitch, they receive a standing ovation from the capacity crowd that no Coventry City team has ever received in its 104-year history. Even the floodlights stand proud, as the crisp night air is penetrated four-fold by their streaming white light. It's a unique moment because the Sky Blues are now semi-finalists in the F. A. Cup, which no City side has previously achieved, despite twenty years in the top flight of English football. This match is just a regular League fixture, but each spectator will be entitled to a voucher for a semi-final ticket in the following month.

It's no normal League match for me, however, as the previous Saturday afternoon I had been at Hillsborough, Sheffield, watching the Sky Blues defeat Sheffield Wednesday 3-1 in the quarter-final to earn their semi-final place. It was the first time I'd seen City win a match in twenty years, as they had been struggling in a football wilderness, while I'd been doing hard labour in a religious wilderness. Now, it seems, destiny is bringing us back together as I rediscover the first love of my childhood and teenage years.

Sitting near to my old season-ticket seat, I'm overawed by the situation as I explain to my friend, Mike: "Mike, it feels like I'm in a twenty-year time warp—and that this place is my real church and my real cathedral. Here are my roots and my long-lost faith—why did I ever go away?"

I'm the Prodigal Son [73] returning home, with the twenty years between 'then' and 'now' collapsed into nothing, as I feel my fractured identity being restored by this single unifying experience. It's good to have Mike to share this with and the match itself ends 3-0 to City. From now on, I shall attend as many matches as I can, home and away, for the rest of the season—and I do.

It was around the time of City's win at Manchester United (3.7) that I first heard Carly Simon's *Coming Around Again* as it climbed the UK charts. It resonated with me at a time when I'd restored some of my pop collection and had been out with a couple of non-religious girlfriends—Francesca and Marie. Could it be that my former pre-religious teenage life was coming around again, now that I had escaped the choking entanglements of religion? But a successful Coventry City again? It seemed like an impossible dream—but a dream that's now becoming increasingly real with every passing game.

*

The sky is blue, the sun is shining and only the chink of a milk bottle in Desolation Row disturbs the geometric rows of terraces from their deep Sunday sleep. I'm catching a breath of early morning air but already I can sense the boiling cauldron of football fervour in four hours' time and just seventy miles away at Hillsborough, with a 12.00 kick-off. It's the F. A. Cup semi-final: *Coventry City* v *Leeds United* for a place in the F. A. Cup Final at Wembley—a place where Leeds had been before, but never Coventry City.

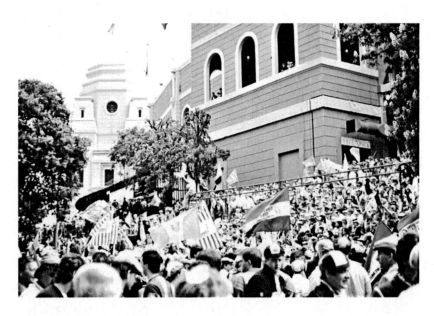

Coventry fans congregate outside Wembley for the greatest day in the club's history

Mike and I leave the car in a Sheffield suburb and walk two miles to the ground, to merge with the masses of Coventry City fans in streams of cars, minibuses, coaches and on foot—all decked out in Sky Blue and white, proceeding in carnival mood towards the Hillsborough stadium. Supporters with banners, flags and scarves together with magazine and hot-dog sellers, all fill the atmosphere with chanting, songs, hooters and familiar aromas.

I notice the arrival of the Lord Mayor of Coventry and commentator, Desmond Lineham—and observe the TV vans with their white satellite dishes and miles of cables, which all add to the occasion. A lone evangelical preacher tells us to prepare for Judgement Day—he needn't worry, for that's exactly what we are doing. Inside the ground, over 51,000 fans bay at each other from all sides: the Leeds fans at the Leppings Lane end, with the Coventry City fans packing the vast Hillsborough Kop—near to which Mike and I are seated. Traffic congestion then delays the kick-off, which ramps up the atmosphere another notch. At last, the ref blows his whistle: Judgement Day has arrived.

From the outset, Leeds are on the front foot and score an early goal, while City miss a host of chances. After half-time, as the minutes tick inexorably by, we wonder if we're going to be left empty-handed. But with only twenty minutes remaining, a Leeds mistake right in front of us allows pint-sized substitute Micky Gynn to score for City in front of the Kop. An explosion of noise bursts over the ground, as the tensions and emotions of over an hour are detonated on a scale I'd never witnessed before. Ten minutes later and Keith Houchen rounds the Leeds goalkeeper to make it 2-1. City fans are momentarily in a Sky Blue Heaven, as one banner proclaims. Agonisingly, Leeds restore parity and extra-time is needed to settle things. Gloriously, City score a final tap-in goal to end up 3-2 winners— but only after some world-class goalkeeping saves by City's Steve Ogrizovic.

The team and management dance jigs of delight in the goalmouth below the massive Kop, as it turns Sky Blue in the time-honoured victory salute of the scarves. The moment starts to sink in: after 104 years of footballing history, Coventry City are finally going to Wembley for the F. A. Cup Final of 1987. For all long-suffering Sky Blue fans, it's beyond their wildest dreams!

"Coventry City at Wembley! Some of them still can't believe it!" declares John Motson for the BBC as the City players are introduced to the Duchess of Kent before the 1987 F. A. Cup Final. Neither can I as, from behind the goal, I sing the traditional *Abide with Me* through tear-filled eyes—after three decades of watching televised Cup Finals at home. But now, I'm there for real!

The atmosphere is less raucous than at the semi-final as City fans are overawed by the historic occasion and stadium with its iconic Twin Towers and the musical pageantry of the Massed Bands of the Royal Marines. We are also awed by our opponents, Tottenham Hotspur, the most successful team in the history of the F. A. Cup competition. Played 7: won 7—a perfect Wembley record! It's the F. A. Cup conquerors, with their international stars like Glenn Hoddle, against the Wembley virgins of Coventry City—and the betting is on Spurs to win as the clear favourites.

This inequality of F. A. Cup history is reinforced after just two minutes when Spurs take the lead and City fans are filled with foreboding about a potential 5 or 6-0 thrashing. Thankfully, the team have no such doubts and within ten minutes, they are back level; although they fall behind again 1-2, just before half-time. But they have played well and we fans can continue to believe.

Then, just after the hour mark, City's winger Dave Bennett receives a pass just below where I am standing. As he shapes to cross the ball into the goalmouth, I swing around and focus my camera on the goal. And then it appears—*the ball in the net*—and I *click*, as 25,000 City fans erupt!

It's 2-2 as Keith Houchen has just scored a spectacular diving header right in front of the massed ranks of City fans; it's the most iconic goal in Coventry City's history—Roy of the Rovers stuff—and from then on, the Sky Blues dominate the game and end up winning 3-2, after a Spurs' own goal in extra-time.

As captain Brian Kilcline receives the F. A. Cup from the Duchess of Kent, the *Sky Blue Song* resounds around Wembley one more time…

Tottenham or Chelsea, United or anyone,
They can't defeat us, we'll fight till the game is won! [74].

*

Coventry city-centre is packed that night, with car horns being sounded everywhere and with everybody and everything coloured Sky Blue, including the city's fountains. The following day, there is an open-top bus parade through the City, with a quarter of a million people, including myself, witnessing this unique event: Coventry City with a major football trophy, achieved with such style and against such mighty opponents.

Less than a year since my post-religious and post-Francesca breakdown in Desolation Row, I have now found a base upon which to rebuild my own authentic life—yet what a wonderful, glorious and passionate way to start this journey of rediscovery!

After so many difficulties, so much mental pain and so much recent heartbreak, my life, it seems, is coming around again.

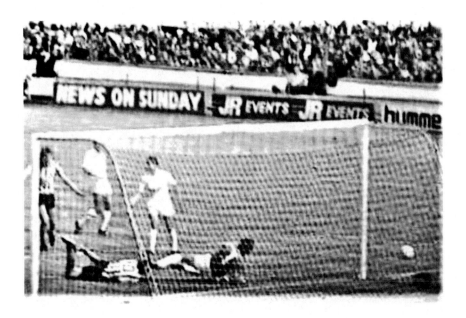

The author's photo of Houchen's iconic equaliser to make it 2-2

4. Moving On

"The thing about you, Jamie, is that you never do anything by halves. Whatever you do, you're always passionate about it."

I'm not sure whether to take Curly's comment as a criticism or a positive endorsement. Perhaps it's just an observation. But nevertheless, it gets me thinking.

The trigger for his comment is my sudden, renewed enthusiasm for Coventry City, following their F. A. Cup success. I had video-recorded the match from both BBC and ITV coverage and had managed to put my own pop music soundtrack to it—songs like *Coming Around Again* and *Live It Up* that caught my mood. I play and replay the video throughout the summer term and holidays—ten minutes each day before I leave for school, as Coventry City once again become part of my spiritual bloodstream. It's the nearest I've got to daily meditation for years!

I go to as many City matches as I possibly can, some with Mike, occasionally with Curly and his son and sometimes with my godson, Ed—a godson from back in my religious years. For Ed's very first match, I manage to get an invitation into the City dressing room and they bring out the F. A. Cup for us to hold. I take a photo of him in his City kit, with a smiling Cyrille Regis sitting behind him [75]. I also start making football scrapbooks. I acquire football magazines and programmes as well as match reports and any articles about the Sky Blues—to cut out the relevant sections and photos and carefully arrange and present them. I also join the Coventry City London Supporters Club—even though I live nowhere near London, so miss out on their weekly meetings and joint travel to Highfield Road and away games. But I receive all their literature and meet some of their characters at away matches. In short, in the twelve months after Wembley, I live, breathe and drink the Sky Blues. No wonder—they've given me my life back.

*

I start to think about things a bit more. I'm intrigued by the twenty-year gap between my support for City in the 1960s and my support now. Why do I feel such a strong identity between my present and my past? Why do I enjoy the strong sense of community with all City supporters, especially at away matches? More specifically, why do I seem to lurch from one 'conversion' experience to another, affected by such powerful, turbulent emotions? First Coventry City, then a conversion to evangelical Christianity, then falling overwhelmingly in love with Francesca—and now it's Coventry City again. What's it all about? *What am I all about?* I have no idea but I continue to think and reflect.

In particular, I wrestle with my identity. I want to ditch the last remnants of a religious identity—the major identity I've had for half my life. I easily get rid of my clerical robes at a local fancy dress shop but it's not so easy getting rid of my inner religious demons. The more I think about my teenage identity—pop music, girls and Coventry City—the happier I am. I'm just a 'Coventry kid' at heart. The problem is that I don't feel like a normal Coventry kid. I don't know of anyone else who's had such a strange, turbulent life. So why am I like this?

I struggle with the feeling that my twenty religious years have been a complete waste of time, when I could have had a far more interesting life enjoying popular culture, socialising and sleeping around. What a wasted life! I'm a mass of confusion and unanswered questions, punctuated with rays of hopeful optimism—such as my return to Coventry City—against a backdrop of pessimism and depression, especially after yet another bad date.

*

As the glory of the F. A. Cup fades, I realise that there are still no girls in football! I miss Francesca all over again. Her empathy, grace and beauty haunt me, and I fear these continued feelings will destroy me. I continue to date attractive, younger women, but none can compare. Most of my meetings are awkward and desperately disappointing. After a wonderful year of football with my newly restored identity, I had felt I was making some progress—for Coventry City feels like therapy. But then I find myself in freefall again. So it's two steps forwards—but three or four steps back. At least, that's how it feels.

'Moving on' might be an illusion. It could be 'moving back' in disguise.

5. Breakout: Chart Therapy
Spring 1989

"Wally, which way?"

"I'm going this way—you go that!"

By now, the guard dogs are out and barking and the searchlights are on. Wally doesn't get very far before he's caught. The other prisoner scampers along the roof, head down. He cuts through some barbed wire and then over the wall, dropping down onto the road below—he's out! For a moment, there's silence, until he hears the guards shouting. Racing through side-streets and across a main road, he disappears into a churchyard where the trees afford some cover. He then trips and slips down a steep slope and into a river, losing a shoe in the process. He swims across the ink-black water without the torchlights spotting him. Dragging himself out, he scrambles up the steep bank and finds himself in college gardens—the gardens of St John's College, Durham! As he lies low in an old outhouse, he's shivering but safe, as he plans his next move.

*

I've just returned home from Coventry after visiting my parents and watching a City match. I flop down in front of the TV and watch whatever's on. I've obviously missed the start of the film, but there's a hole in a prison cell wall the inmates are covering up with papier-mâché. As if in real life, prisoners could make a hole in a wall and cover it up each night with papier-mâché! What a ridiculous plot! It's just not credible.

I then notice the guards' Geordie accents and there's a reference to Mr Callaghan as Home Secretary, and I start to wonder if the film might actually be based on a true story. I continue to be gripped by the breakout when I suddenly realise: it's the escape from Durham Prison that I had got caught up in during my first term in Durham! (2.4) I'm glued till the end—and the eventual recapture of

John McVicar (played by Roger Daltrey) [76]. I'm mesmerised by such a dramatic portrayal of a forgotten past. I'd not thought about Durham since the day I left. Nevertheless, the most significant moment for me is still to come, and it will change my life, again!

*

McVicar was rearrested in London at gunpoint, and there the film ends. For me, however, the action is just about to start as I read the film's post-script, which explains that McVicar was re-arrested in 1970 and received an extended sentence. In jail, he enrolled as an external student of sociology at London University, for which he achieved a first class Honours degree. Then early parole and a return to law-abiding civilian life as a successful journalist and broadcaster.

By sheer coincidence, I had just started studying for a Master's degree in sociology at Nottingham University (5.2) and my brain goes into overdrive, making all sorts of connections:

- McVicar had been to Durham. *I had been to Durham*—contemporaries, for a few weeks.
- McVicar had been in prison. *I had been in a prison*—of religious struggle and doubt.
- I had witnessed the aftermath of McVicar's escape at St John's College.
- His criminal career had subsequently been transformed, through studying sociology.
- My school career is being transformed, through studying and teaching sociology.

I come to focus on three overwhelming thoughts:

1. *I now know of one other person who had experienced a bad time in Durham—and escaped!*
2. *If he could escape, then so can I—escape from my negative feelings about my time in Durham!*
3. *Sociology is obviously a great subject for an escapee!*

I begin to feel liberated and exhilarated, though I'm not sure why. Eventually, the penny drops: it's the first time in eighteen years that I've admitted to having had an awful time in Durham! I had arrived there with such high hopes: of a warm evangelical college, where I would grow in the Christian faith and leave as a second Billy Graham—well, maybe! But it had just taken a few months in Durham for this fantasy to come crashing down—through the Sargant lecture—and then later through the shock of Celia breaking off our engagement. In truth, the disillusionment had been so great that I had simply 'buried' it when I left—it was all too painful to contemplate.

When I next see Maggie, her reaction to my story is one of complete surprise: "You've been coming to me for counselling for four years, yet you've never mentioned Durham once! It's obviously something you've seriously repressed."

*

Discovering Chart Therapy

Feeling relieved of a great burden that I never knew I had (certainly at a conscious level), I'm keen to express my discovery in some way—but how?

I get a piece of squared A4 paper, 33 squares wide and 22 squares high. Using the 22 squares as my *vertical* axis, I draw a horizontal line half-way down. This will give me 2 squares for a title, plus 10 'positive' squares above the mid-line, graded +1 to +10. Similarly -1 to -10 'negative' squares below. For the *horizontal* axis, each square represents a year, from 1960-90, which I label. I then start to colour in those years that have significant highs or lows. For example, 1969, the year of the Sargant lecture was an extremely bad year, therefore I score it as -9. So I colour in 9 squares below the mid-line (in dark brown) for that year. On the other hand, 1987 was absolutely brilliant, with Coventry City winning the F. A. Cup, so I score it +10 and colour that year in, all 10 squares above the mid-line— in Sky Blue, of course. In the large areas of blank squares, I place three photos: Durham Cathedral as a negative, below the mid-line; and of Francesca and Coventry City as positives, above. It's rough, it's crude, it's basic—but it's a form of confession (to myself) of both the very bad, as well as the very good, years. It feels as therapeutic as any session with Maggie. It's the start of what I call *Chart Therapy*.

Exhilarated by both the content and the creative process, other charts follow on all aspects of my life to date. I swiftly move on to the charting of all the football grounds I've been to supporting the Sky Blues—32 so far. Then a multicoloured dart-shaped chart, which I call *The Reconstruction of Identity*. Some charts are merely lists—of pop music, TV programmes, friends and disasters (both personal and national). All of them uncover aspects of my past life that has been clouded by two decades of religious adherence and psychological angst. But now, these years are coming back to life—to be remembered, celebrated or mourned—and I'm starting to feel alive again! There's also a list of all the young ladies I've encountered over my forty years of life, from childhood crushes to a long-term, live-in relationship. For this, there are twenty names, which I find both impressive *and* depressing: too much quantity, not enough quality! Over the next few years, I produce nearly a hundred such charts, all carefully hand-coloured and scattered throughout with relevant photos to illustrate the bar-charts and other statistics that are presented.

I find that chart therapy is both creative *and* reflective. It's confessional *and* celebratory. It shines a mirror on my life and helps me recover lost memories. I also leave spaces for the future on my charts—a future that would soon be witnessing another sort of breakout as, later that year, the Berlin Wall comes down.

My own Berlin Wall, at the end of Desolation Row, remains unmoved—but fortunately, I have now gathered enough finances to move to a better part of town…as my own personal and therapeutic breakout continues.

Errata
p164 line 11 should read: *two* years not four years.
p390 line 9 (Note 139) should read: 'attachment *dis*order'.
p394 Further Reading **add**: Machin A. (2022) '*Why We Love*', esp. Ch.3 & 8.

6. Thinking Straight

I'm standing outside the Nottingham Playhouse, waiting for a date—a hot date!

I've talked to Debbie several times on the phone and she's very flirty! We've written letters and exchanged photos, and she looks and sounds beautiful! I'm very excited and I really hope that we might get together pretty soon—it's a long time since I had so much as a hug!

I check my watch. I've been daydreaming about Debbie, and she's five minutes late. No matter. She'll be here soon—we've got to know each other so well over the past few weeks. She won't let me down…I hope.

I check my watch again. She's 15 minutes late, and I can feel my stomach tightening and my anxiety rising. I need a hug more than ever, but am I going to get one when I need it so much?

After 30 minutes, I'm close to despair—am I being stood up? I've had lots of dates before, but I've never been stood up. How can anyone do such a thing? She could have phoned me!

After 40 minutes, I give up. I'm gutted. There must be an explanation. When I get home, I'll phone her and it will be all sorted out—either that or I'll let her know *exactly* how I feel!

Once home, I'm on the phone straightaway. It's engaged—and remains engaged for the twenty times I redial throughout the evening. I eventually conclude that I have been stood up. I'm devastated. Has she got no manners, no courtesy, no respect for my feelings? No basic human decency? I'm beyond angry!

First thing in the morning, I phone again—a dialling tone at last! But Debbie gets in first: "Fuck off! I've met someone else!" And she puts the phone down.

That was my lovely, flirty, beautiful Debbie! I'm incandescent with rage—so I arrange to see my therapist, Maggie.

*

Maggie is sympathetic, though not very empathetic towards my plight. By the time the session is over, I've learnt that my anger and despair is mainly my fault and not Debbie's! This is often the case with Maggie, when I feel that I've been let down by someone else.

To start with, Maggie suggests that I have engaged in *fantastical thinking* about Debbie—before ever meeting her—which only heightens my expectations. It's fair point, I suppose. Also, Maggie suggests that I have a *low frustration threshold,* an *inflexible demanding philosophy* and prone to *awfulizing* situations. In other words, although being stood up on a date is disappointing, it is not, in fact, the end of the world.

"Jamie, how many times have you been stood up on your dates? And do you suppose that other people get stood up too—or is it only you?"

Sheepishly, I reply that this was my first time and that other people, I suppose, get stood up too.

"In which case, I suggest that you have fared better than average, and that you're no different from other people who have also been stood up, or who have been treated badly in other ways."

I arrive back home, a bit down but having lost my feelings of despair. According to Maggie, I've been engaged in *unrealistic thinking*, with various *cognitive distortions* making things worse. By which she means that I am not actually the centre of the universe and there is no law to say that other people will always behave as I'd like them to. I've been given my first difficult lesson in *cognitive therapy*—and it wouldn't be the last. In fact, things do get much, much worse before I start to learn how to think straight for myself.

*

Unlike Debbie, Penny is a very real person. Tall, blonde and athletic, she's in the women's 'A' team at my local tennis club, which I've joined for the summer season. Due to others' holiday absences, I manage to make it into the men's 'B' team for a few matches. On club nights, however, during the long summer evenings, Penny and I often pair up against other couples to play some friendly mixed-doubles.

Off court, we get chatting about relationships and in particular about her recent rejection from a high-voltage love affair that she had hoped was leading to something permanent. She's aware that I've had my own fair share of rejections, and I'm an empathetic listener. Moreover, I reckon I can help her best if I identify fully with her pain and 'merge' my own traumatic experiences with hers. For several months, we meet regularly to talk about our respective traumas—well into the chilly autumn. Eventually, on one particularly cold evening, we merge our bodies as well as our souls. It's been a long time since I've enjoyed skin-to-skin contact and I'm optimistic about the prospect of more.

However, that never happens as Penny, quite unexpectedly, withdraws from me and distances herself both physically and emotionally. The parting is sudden. No farewell kiss or even a hug as I leave. Just when some warmth, affection and sex seemed to be available, it's immediately withdrawn—and I've no idea why. It feels like the sharpest of rejections. I'm at a loss—and feeling lost once more, as my emotions start to spiral downwards.

By the time December arrives, I've run out of dates. Indeed, I had stopped dating while seeing Penny, expecting a happier Christmas than usual. But now I'm alone and lonely and in freefall—heading into a bottomless chasm. I don't want to be here! I don't want to live this horrendous life! So I decide to play Russian roulette by running a red light at a major crossroads, to let fate decide whether I live or die. En route to the crossroads, I spy a young couple with their arms around each other and looking into each other's eyes, and I know for certain that this will never happen to me again—even if I live.

As green and amber turn to red, I press the accelerator hard. Then, in a split second, I think of little Ed, my godson, sweet and innocent and tucked up in bed—and press hard on the brake pedal. The car lurches and screeches to a stop in the middle of the crossroads. Car horns blare at me, but happily there's no articulated lorry to finish me off. I make my way sheepishly into a side street and pull up. I've just given myself the fright of my life!

I'm still shaking as I drive myself back home, wondering what to do—how to do *something* to relieve my pain. I trawl through the entertainment section of a local magazine and spot an advert for a strip-club. I head over there—it's my first time and a new experience. I'm not allowed to touch, I know that, but I can *see*, and that alone might give me a boost. I'm not brave enough to slip a fiver into Roxy's thong as she performs her routine but after she's got her clothes back on, I pluck up the courage to have a chat with her at the bar, whilst other men keep their distance, as if in awe. She seems pleased to have someone to talk to, though I limit myself to ten minutes, then prepare to leave.

"Jamie, it's been nice talking to you. You take care, sweetheart"—before pressing her lips to my cheek and giving me a friendly farewell hug.

I return home, soothed by her kindness and still feeling her kiss. In a mirror, I examine the lipstick imprint on my face and slowly but surely, my pain ebbs away.

*

Once again, I turn to Maggie and tell her the story in some detail. She listens thoughtfully before commenting: "First of all, trying to *merge* with Penny was not a good idea, because I think you were actually trying to deal with your own needs, not just hers. And being rejected, when you had put so much of yourself into the relationship, was bound to be more painful than if you'd kept yourself more separate. As for the young couple you saw, you were *catastrophizing* about them—blowing things out of all proportion, due to your negative emotional state. Your Russian roulette is, of course, very serious. I think you must have been experiencing the *cognitive triad*" [77].

"Go on…"

"The cognitive triad is when:

1. you feel bad about yourself, for example, you feel unlovable
2. when you feel the world is against you, or, as in your case, when you feel that women are against you
3. when you can't see anything changing in the future

"It seems that all these things were going on in your head in a vicious circle. Thankfully, your godson gave you a glimmer of positivity…and so did Roxy, of course," she added with a wry smile.

"But what did I get so wrong about Penny?"

"Well, try to reframe the situation. Just think—she's just come out of a huge love-affair, similar to you and Francesca. After Francesca, what happened to the girl next door, Marie?"

"I didn't want her, because I was still in love with Francesca."

"Precisely. Don't you see? Penny's rejection is not actually about you—it's about her own loss—and your brief success in getting close to her made her feel that loss ever more keenly."

169

"You mean, I caught Penny on the rebound? And because I merged with her, her rejection felt even worse—because she was still in love with her ex?"

"That's what it looks like to me."

"You mean I went through hell because I caught someone on the rebound? Why didn't I see that—it's so obvious—*now*!"

"But it's not going to be obvious when your thinking is so clouded by your own emotional needs and *that's* where your problem lies."

*

I learnt a lot from Maggie in these sessions about how to think straight. Thankfully, my escapade with Penny was to be the lowest point of my post-religious, rollercoaster experience, which was, in essence, nothing to do with Penny but everything to do with my poor understanding and handling of the situation. Maggie was also proved right about my catastrophic thinking about the young couple. For only a few months later, I became involved with Millie and started enjoying affection and love once more (3.8).

7. Script Analysis
Autumn 1992

"So then Jamie, for you it was a choice between Cinderella and Goldilocks and the Three Bears? Explain."

*

I'm travelling home with Maggie from a day-conference on Script Analysis [78], organised for her post-graduate students. It's good to chat informally with her, for once.

"But why Cinderella?" she continued. "It's usually *women* who identify with Cinderella, as several did today."

"Cinderella needed saving by Prince Charming—and if I were gay, then Prince Charming would be fine—but as I'm not, then I need a *Princess* Charming to save me."

"Go on..."

"As far back as I can remember, since my childhood romance with Glenda at junior school (1.3), I've wanted a warm, affectionate, romantic lady in my life to fill the empty space inside. I seem lost without such a lady—or at least without the possibility of finding her."

Maggie remains thoughtful at the steering wheel.

"I think this need goes back to what you didn't get from your mother. Even so, you've not done too badly: you had four years with Celia, then Holly and a much longer relationship with Sophie."

"But all those were limited or spoiled by religion. I need a non-religious girlfriend now."

"But since then, you've met Francesca and Millie—and now Karla—who are all non-religious." (3.6-9)

"But it doesn't last—I always get rejected! And with Karla, it's not romantic, it's just sex and friendship."

Maggie seems concerned that I want to put all my eggs into one basket—the basket of exclusive, unending, romantic love and that such thinking does indeed make me like Cinderella—dependent on an external source for what (I think) I need, and over which I have no control.

"It makes you a hostage to fortune, James, and very vulnerable. But I actually think you are doing much better than that… Let me explain."

*

The conference had opened with Maggie asking us all to try to identify a 'script' from childhood. In other words, a strong message received in childhood, from parents or any other source, that resonates with us and our life story at an emotional level. Other sources may be dreams, fantasies and fairy-tales. Once decided upon, we were each asked to share them with the group.

I couldn't identify a specific 'script' from my parents, so I went for a childhood fairy-story. Several women in the group identified with *Cinderella*, which I had thought about myself, but my first choice was *Goldilocks and the Three Bears*—mainly because I identified with Baby Bear, whose bowl of porridge Goldilocks had eaten and whose chair she had broken. I felt a bit like that—all my attempts at romance had been eaten up and the four-square gospel of evangelical Christianity had had all its legs broken, leaving me with nothing. It's a sad story—Coventry City notwithstanding—and it's certainly the way I tended to look at my life.

*

Maggie has other ideas however, which she explains as we continue homewards in her car.

"Jamie, I'm not persuaded about your empty bowl of porridge. In fact, I reckon you've got several bowls full of porridge all lined up! Just think about what you *have* and what you have *achieved* in the years I've known you."

Intrigued, I ask her to explain.

"Jamie, since leaving religion behind, you've enjoyed several valuable relationships from which you've learnt a lot, and I happen to think that Karla is very good for you too. You have a positive relationship with Ed, you're deeply interested in sociology, especially with your Nottingham MA (5.2) and you've even introduced Transactional Analysis into your school (5.4). You've gained some more friends through school and Coventry City—and you're having fun through your reborn interest in pop, football, scrapbooks and chart-making. You have a lot going on and most of it is positive. Moreover, you are starting to nurture *yourself*, instead of depending on other people all the time. No one has to be stuck with their childhood script, including you. You can change it—and it seems to me that you've already started."

*

As Maggie drops me off at home, my head is spinning. I hadn't thought about my post-religious life like that before. So, after the football results and tea, I take another sheet of A4 paper and gather my pencil, pencil crayons and a coin to draw round, for some porridge bowls!

For I feel another chart—a more positive chart—coming on.

8. Catharsis

At the end of the 50s, Connie Francis was singing about 'Lipstick on Your Collar' [79] that told a tale of a husband's infidelity. Before long, it would unleash many more tales from my half-remembered childhood.

*

One side-effect of my chart-therapy was that I had started to investigate my pre-religious past, now that my repression about my time in Durham had been uncovered and acknowledged. My teenage life in the swinging Sky Blue sixties was not difficult to recall as it had been such a colourful and dramatic decade—whether from Sky Blue success, pulsating pop, politics, Profumo, the Cold War or England's 1966 World Cup victory. The memories even stretched back to spring 1959 and my first visit to Highfield Road. But what came *before* Coventry City? A bit like asking what came before the Big Bang! Nothing—at least nothing to talk of. Just the very grey and foggy 1950s.

But all that was about to change when, in February 1993, Mike comes around to my place to watch Dennis Potter's screenplay, *Lipstick On Your Collar* [80]. It's in six weekly parts, so we're in for the long haul…

The early scenes at the War Office, where battle plans are being drawn up for the invasion of Suez (1956) are somewhat tedious. I'd rather see more of the gorgeous Sylvia Berry—a beauty in her early twenties, with tumbling golden hair, rosy red lips, swinging hips and a polka-dot skirt. She's sweet and kind with a winning smile and a twinkle in her eye. The introverted, stuttering Private Francis, a fellow lodger, is in awe of her and would love to snatch a kiss—and so would I!

Sylvia is an usherette at her local cinema for a few evenings a week 'to make ends meet', but on a Saturday evening, she's off to the Hammersmith Palais to dance the night away. The funny thing is that I feel that I've met her before somewhere, but I've not the faintest idea where or when.

She's a bit sweet on Private Francis, attracted by his gentle manner, and they manage to have an awkward fumble one afternoon, while her bully of a husband is away. Outside their cheap bedsit, all is quiet. A single black Austin car is parked down the street; children play hopscotch by the crumbling red-brick wall; and a couple of housewives in curlers and headscarves clean their windows and wash their steps. The funny thing is, I feel I've been here before as well—but again, I can't think where or when. I've a strong sense of déjà vu.

The music of the 50s inserts itself into every scene, including the War Office, with Private Hopper (Ewan McGregor) jumping on his desk at one point and rocking along to *Blue Suede Shoes*—in his fantasies at least. I know all the songs, for that's when 'pop' started for me in the late 50s with Elvis, Rock 'n' Roll, Bill Haley and Buddy Holly, as precious memories start to stir.

*

I'm totally absorbed by *Lipstick* and by the time the series ends, I've had another revelation: I realise that the street scene outside Sylvia's lodgings is where Spot the dog chased me (1.2), the Hammersmith Palais is where I met the girls who helped me dance (1.5) and Sylvia is, of course, Auntie Caroline—warm, sweet, loveable, kind and deliciously naughty! (1.4) At last, I'm starting to uncover some important people and events from my earliest years.

During the series, I receive a letter from my MA tutor at Nottingham, and suddenly, I've a decision to make. The letter encourages me to apply for an M. Litt on the basis of a recent, long essay that I've sent him: *The Sociology of Emotion* (5.3). I'm very flattered and sorely tempted. However, I sense a greater desire forming within me—a desire to write about my emotions—now that *Lipstick* has unlocked the 1950s for me, and with it, my childhood. So I forgo the higher degree in order to follow my heart—for I want to write out the stories that have given me my life.

I start to write in early April and I don't stop till late June, exhausted. I write these autobiographical stories in the early morning, waking myself up at 2 am. And I continue with them after school and into the evening. At some point, I must have done some schoolwork! It seems that *Lipstick* has unlocked my early life—just as *McVicar* had unlocked my 'prison' experience in Durham. Both these film events feel extremely valuable, fulfilling and therapeutic.

*

The first story I write is about my first sensuous encounter with Sophie (3.4). Then many more stories come tumbling out, in any order and from any decade—like a rushing stream cascading down a steep and rocky valley. Throughout this outpouring of my life-story, I see Karla every month (3.9), who's fascinated and impressed by this, my latest project.

"I must say, Jamie, you don't do anything by halves, do you?"

Karla takes my stories back home with her to read and returns them the following month with her observations, comments, questions and positive support. It's the most wonderful kind of therapy. By late June, I'm exhausted from writing, having got over 40 stories out of my system. More will follow later.

Eventually, I stop writing—and immediately fall into depression for a couple of weeks and wonder what's going on. I soon realise that it's the result of sleep deprivation, from which I quickly recover. I then enter into a flat calm, a sort of Nirvana, where a 'still centre' prevails. For I've been striving all my life to cope with varied threats to my emotional well-being. Now, at last, I'm at peace. It's an eerie, strange, new feeling, which a song that I've recently heard captures well. For Abba's *When All Is Said and Done* [81] speaks to me of being calm at the crossroads of life, having lost the need to be continually striving, looking for oneself. It fits me perfectly. Karla thinks that I should get my stories published, but I'm not so sure. They are too raw, rough and ready for my liking and not reflective enough. But I collect them into their chronological sequence, despite some important gaps. The title seems obvious enough: *Living with Passion.*

*

Amid all my emotional outpourings, however, one reflection stands out crystal clear: that I get easily and passionately attached to both people and institutions—Coventry City, evangelical religion, Celia, Francesca, Millie—and almost every other lady with whom I get beyond a first date. It's a near continuous and emotionally exhausting rollercoaster, although my present relationship with Karla is different and feels like a big improvement. But I want to understand *why* I get so easily attached and why I don't know anyone else who seems to be like me. Skimming through my TV magazine for the following week, I see a programme on precisely this theme—so I sit up and take notice!

176

9. Attachment Theory
December 1993

There's a film clip of a disturbed young man in mental hospital. Then of women at work in a factory during World War II. Followed by mother and child in the Strange Situation [82].

Finally, an elderly man in a deerstalker talks to the camera: "Maternal love is just like vitamins. Without vitamins, you don't get physical health, and without maternal love, you don't get mental health."

*

The man in the deerstalker is John Bowlby, the co-founder of Attachment Theory with Mary Ainsworth, whose 'Strange Situation' experiment has become one of the most frequently used research tools in psychology. These and the earlier scenes are from the 30-minute film: *Are Mothers Really Necessary?* [83] I had started to realise the importance of the early years of childhood ever since my relationship with Millie (3.8), but with this short film, interest was turning into conviction. Bowlby went on to say that: "An infant should experience a warm, intimate and continuous relationship with his mother (or mother-substitute) in which both find satisfaction and enjoyment." [84] That sounds good and how it should be, but it's totally outside of my experience. It seems I had suffered from maternal deprivation [85] and perhaps explains why Maggie had asked me about my mother in our first counselling session, which had so enraged me (4.1). I now want to know more—a lot more!

I scour Nottingham university bookshop for anything about Attachment, before discovering the perfect volume: *John Bowlby and Attachment Theory* by Jeremy Holmes, published earlier that year [86]. I read it all in a few days, making notes and underlining sections all the way through. In particular, I write down a list of the difficulties I had experienced with my parents in those early years, focussing on my mother's trauma and depression and the inadequacy of the substitute care provided. By the time I'm finished, I feel that I understand myself in a way that I never have before. My life *makes sense* now—the good, the bad and the ugly—and it brings a great deal of relief. Perhaps there are still some t's to be crossed and i's to be dotted—but I believe that Attachment Theory will last me a lifetime. After the Gospel of Coventry City and the Gospel of Jesus Christ, it's now the Gospel of Attachment Theory! Among the key ideas that resonate with me are the following:

a. The maternal deprivation I suffered, happened at about twelve months old—precisely the age when an infant's attachment bonds are forming, so it's not surprising that I was seriously affected.

b. This deprivation was through inconsistent parenting, which generated anxiety within me. Will I get the cuddles and love I want and need? Or will I be turned away, isolated and alone?

c. I realise that I am anxiously-ambivalently attached—as all the descriptors in Holmes' book point in that direction—and none in the direction of a secure or avoidant attachment.

d. I also realise why I feel so alone in my anxious-ambivalence because, in Ainsworth's original (USA) study, only 12% are ambivalently attached. In UK studies, they remain the smallest group at 15%; with avoidantly attached 20%; and securely attached 65% of the population. I'm overjoyed to learn that there *are* others like me, although it's a fairly small minority—I'm not alone! And it may explain why I've not met anyone that's similar to me—there aren't that many of us!

e. Bowlby's 'internal working model' that children develop when young seems to apply to me, as my childhood difficulties persisted through adolescence and into adulthood, and I continue to act and react in passionate and sometimes extreme ways.

f. My romantic 'style' also matches the descriptors for the ambivalently attached [87], being very needy, clingy and wanting to 'merge' with the beloved, which often drives partners away. I'm also anxious about being abandoned, which can become a self-fulfilling prophecy.

g. I often experience acute separation-anxiety when I'm physically or emotionally distant from my latest partner. I experience *chronic vigilance* for signs of a partner about to abandon me. And then *chronic grief* when they do so. It is the latter that Maggie immediately sensed when I first went to see her about Francesca (3.7 & 4.1). All of these negative feelings are particularly associated with being anxious-ambivalently attached, although not exclusively so.

*

Typically, I'm in a rush to enthuse with anyone who will listen to my new Gospel. Maggie is my first audience, which includes a rant about my parents and how much I want to visit them to tell them exactly what I think about them. Maggie's reply is judicious and wise, as always: "I'd really think twice about that, Jamie, for it would have effects beyond what you want. Certainly, you'd get some feelings off your chest. But it would further damage your relationship with your parents who, in other respects, have brought you up really well. They too were victims of their own circumstances, just as you have been. And it was you who chose to get into religion, not them."

Points taken, I hurry home with my tail between my legs—and not for the first time. Clearly, I still have a great deal to learn.

In the months that follow my 'discovery' of Attachment Theory, I feel a lot calmer. I deal with Karla's departure after Christmas with equanimity and I don't feel the need to rush back immediately into more dating. When I do, it's less frenetic than before. When I'm disappointed by a date, I don't find myself 'grieving' as much, and inwardly, I don't feel so lonely, even when I'm alone, which is most of the time when I'm not at school. My 'highs' are not as manic and my 'lows' are not so despairing. Internally, my psychological world seems to be changing—but slowly. I can still get my knickers in a twist over this or that lady who doesn't respond to me in the way that I'd like. I can forgive myself that—for underneath my emerging feelings of inner security, I accept that, at root, I'm still anxious-ambivalently attached and will sometimes over-react.

*

While my internal world is undergoing a gradual, although uneven, transformation, events are also starting to move in my external world of work. Two years later at school, the Head invites me into his study for coffee.

"James. Good to see you. How do you like your coffee? Black or white? Sugar? I've asked you to come here because I've recently received a petition from twenty Year 11 students, all very bright. Here's their petition. Have a read and tell me what you think."

Actually, I'm aware that this petition would be coming (see 5.3-4) but I don't let on—at least, not yet.

I'm much more interested in Mr Milburn's reaction—will he approve or dismiss it out of hand?

I hold my breath.

10. Therapies: Review

There were two driving forces behind my eight years of intense therapy in 1986-93: the input of Maggie's psychotherapy and the output of my own self-therapy. Both were essential for my eventual recovery. Not that recovery was complete by the end of 1993—far from it. But the railway lines of psychotherapy and self-therapy proved themselves adequate to keep my recovery on track and to prevent me going off the rails or hitting the buffers. My therapeutic journey was aided by two strokes of considerable good fortune: the competency and generosity of Maggie as my therapist, and the timing of Coventry City's F. A. Cup success, which facilitated my return to that first secure attachment and clear identity of my pre-religious years (1.6).

On this matter, John Bowlby's view was: "the human psyche is strongly inclined towards self-healing. The psychotherapist's job is to provide the conditions in which self-healing can best take place." [88]

This supports my view that, without the skill and commitment of the therapist and *the active engagement* of one's self, the therapy train will not even leave the station.

A. Psychotherapy

i. Unless one is raised in a household where therapy is accepted and talked about as a part of modern life, the most difficult step for a person in crisis is the first one—as that involves an admission of need and often an admission of the failure of one's own efforts hitherto. Personally, I found it utterly humiliating to admit that I needed a counsellor at all. For the uninitiated, it's a call to be courageous in the face of the unknown. It's unlikely to be an easy ride; there may be dark tunnels to enter that you

181

didn't see coming, as well as shafts of insight that inspire you to continue your journey in hope.

For me, there were three such tunnels: anything to do with my mother; my feelings of social isolation; and, worst of all, the turning of the spotlight on myself when all I wanted was Maggie's collusion in blaming other people for having let me down. *That* was difficult to stomach, but stomach it I did, and I emerged from the other end with a much greater sense of control.

ii. Maggie was wise in not pursuing my 'mother' issue head on: perhaps she sensed that I might leave therapy altogether. However, through Transactional Analysis (TA), my relationships with my mother, and Sophie, could be explored more obliquely. Yet it was I who had raised TA terms such as 'critical parent' and 'free child' in the first place. Maggie was more than happy to go with my flow—and so the development of TA as part of the therapy was a genuinely interactive conversation that, in time, would become an important part of my future.

iii. Maggie's introduction of *Rational Emotive Therapy* in dealing with my affair with Penny, and my being stood up, was immensely helpful in getting me to see that it was my own assumptions and interpretation of events that left me in such a forlorn state on both occasions. By thinking differently, I could have processed and handled both situations differently and with far less inner turmoil. I learnt my lesson for, in the years that followed, I found myself able to navigate similar tricky waters with greater control and equanimity, as I no longer turned disappointments into disasters. However, all the 'straight thinking' in the world cannot fill the empty space in one's soul. It's only one's inner attachments that can fill these empty spaces (section *B*).

iv. Spotting Millie's unconscious *Uproar* game (3.8) was very important for me, especially as I find it hard to understand most of Berne's other 'Games' due to not having experienced them myself—or at least, not being aware that I have. I appreciated Maggie's willingness to see Millie and myself together, for it was from that meeting and subsequent discussions with Millie that I was able to piece together her psychological history. The process was self-therapy as much as it was Millie-therapy, as in many ways we were similar; I was continuing to develop insights into my own life and, as a result, I started to become less reliant on Maggie.

v.   My introduction by Maggie to Script Analysis also proved worthwhile, due to her understanding of my journey so far and her positive reinterpretation of my Baby Bear story with his empty porridge bowl. I did not pursue Script Analysis further as it did not resonate with me like the primary aspects of TA had done. I didn't want or need any more theory—just application, which I could do for myself through my Chart Therapy work.

vi. Maggie had provided me with a safe haven that afforded me some protection after Francesca had left—and a secure base in which I could place my trust for my therapeutic journey into unknown territory. These are the two main functions of a secure attachment. In therapy, Maggie had become a temporary attachment figure for me and, as such, had provided a secure base function for the time I was in therapy and beyond. I could call upon her any time in the following years, when I encountered emotional turbulence I couldn't understand. According to Jeremy Holmes [89], this provision of a secure base function is the hallmark of a therapist's role—a role Maggie had performed exceptionally well.

B. Self-therapy

i.   If asked to select one single factor that promoted my recovery in Desolation Row and beyond, it would have to be Coventry City's winning of the F. A. Cup in 1987. Indeed, it's a close-run thing between Cup Final magic and Maggie, which together provided a perfect combination: re-attachment to the first (institutional) love of my teenage years and Maggie who facilitated my ongoing therapeutic journey. My re-attachment to the Sky Blues and my restored identity was the healing itself; whereas the focus with Maggie was talking about healing [90]. In the longer view, however, Maggie's therapy proved more useful as it taught me ways of being and relating that I could never learn from Coventry City, however successful they were.

ii. Other aspects of my re-attachment to Coventry City are also significant—especially the fact that I had no knowledge of Attachment Theory at the time. Therefore, my 'Aha' moment when I returned to Highfield Road after thirteen years (4.3) was a raw, spontaneous and heartfelt reaction. The reconnection was emotional rather than theoretical: it was a massive welcoming party for my homecoming to the secure base of my pre-religious teenage years.

My enjoyment of City's success also felt more intimate than during the years of my teenage support. Previously, I had always had a sense of 'something missing' as a teenager, and now I didn't, following the rediscovery of a deeper self through Francesca and Maggie. Furthermore, for most of the matches I attended that year, I had Mike as a companion. I could talk to Mike about everything going on inside me—and in the world—and not just about football. Together, these factors made my experiences of 1987 far richer, deeper and heart-warming than my earlier teenage experience.

However, as all football fans know, there is always a downside to supporting a particular club. In attachment terms, Coventry City Football Club is *reliable*, in that it always exists [91], but it is not always *consistent* in the quality of what it offers. Neither had it improved in meeting my needs for a social life, especially with 60 miles of geographical distance between Coventry and Grantham. My underlying attachment, especially since the F. A. Cup run of 1987 was strong, but my actual commitment has fluctuated according to the team's success, or the lack of it. At the height of 1987 though, and for a few years beyond, the club had restored my first secure identity since the dark days of a lost faith and failed relationships with Sophie and Francesca. Both literally and figuratively, I had, at last, something to sing about!

iii. If my re-attachment to Coventry City was a bolt from the blue, my discovery of Chart Therapy was a projectile from prison: explosive and painful, blasting through my defences and releasing new energy into my psychological awareness. My identification with the *McVicar* TV experience of 'escaping imprisonment in Durham' first shook me to the core, then propelled the therapeutic process onto a different plane. From then on, I dared look at anything and everything in my past and present life—to confess, analyse, measure, objectify and ultimately accept or even celebrate—and in the process, discover and develop an imaginative, creative side to myself, which proved immensely fulfilling.

iv. My subsequent story-telling as a cathartic response to the *Lipstick* series, unlocking my '50s childhood, was in effect the verbalisation of Chart Therapy, but with another decade to pore over and with greater emotional nuancing than is possible with charts. I see the charts as structured visualisations of the stories that, in that form, are easier to grasp. I continue to use both processes today: I write stories and I draw charts—they are the diet-and-exercise of my psychological well-being. They help me enjoy being myself (most of the time) and have kept me (relatively) sane for the past thirty years.

v. Without the recollection of my 1950s childhood memories, I would never have understood and adopted Attachment Theory as fully as I did at the end of 1993. Those memories (1.2-1.5) together with my mother's oft-repeated story of *The Unforgettable Night* (1.1) now made perfect sense to me as I came to realise how well Attachment Theory applied to me. I was fortunate that, back in the 1990s, I could see myself as anxious-ambivalently attached without any doubt or qualification. I was the stereotypical model for ambivalence, in the Attachment meaning of the word. Psychologically speaking, it's not a good place to be. But at least I knew where (and who) I was, which was a great deal better than being entirely lost in a religious fog. Attachment theory was the hat that fitted and I was happy to wear it, although today I would identify as having some 'earned security' through autobiographical competence (3.10iv) as I increased in self-understanding and awareness.

vi. There are however some important qualifications to make. Although in 1993, I could easily self-identify as ambivalently attached, I strongly suspect I was among a small minority who could readily identify with a specific attachment status. This is for three main reasons:

1. Those securely and avoidantly attached will not feel the need to investigate their childhood roots or attachment status, although for quite different reasons [92].

2. Recent Attachment research has suggested that security, avoidance and ambivalence are better viewed as aspects of a flexible attachment continuum, rather than fixed attachment types. In other words, while some people may self-identify with one particular type, the majority will not. For them, they may feel, for example, a mixture of ambivalence and avoidance, or ambivalence but with some 'earned' security. Even the earliest researchers accepted that one can have a different attachment type with a different person, e.g., with different parents. Therefore, most people will find it difficult to self-identify with a clear-cut type.

3. Sir Michael Rutter's critique of Bowlby and the longitudinal *Minnesota Study* [93] have provided strong evidence that, for many, other social-psychological concerns outweigh the importance of underlying attachments. Such concerns include, for example: a severely disrupted home-life; serious physical and/or sexual abuse; post-traumatic stress or other severe mental health problems; unwanted pregnancy and alcohol, drug and other addictions. While underlying attachment issues predispose individuals to better (or worse) outcomes, it is accepted that in such situations, the main factor that needs addressing is the problematic behaviour itself and its immediate roots. Sometimes, attachment issues need to take a backseat in counselling and therapy.

If my experiences with Coventry City and with Maggie's counselling sessions were the therapeutic railway tracks that guided my post-religious life, then Attachment Theory was the major railway interchange to which these tracks inevitably led.

After arriving at this destination, the importance of my football club and Maggie's therapy tended to retract, now that their therapeutic tasks were more or less complete. Attachment Theory itself became my secure base as, along with my continuing stories and charts, it provided me with a considerable degree of autobiographical competence. In other words, I can make psychological sense of my own life-story. This in turn provides me with "my own internal secure base"

[94]. Desirable as such a development may be, it comes with a very serious health warning: *Attachment security offers no guarantee of avoiding future major crises!* In the years that will follow (5.4 onwards), I will encounter that painful truth for myself, again and again.

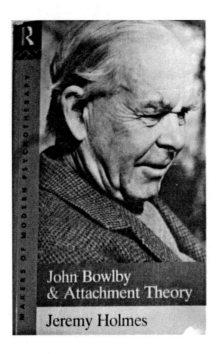

The book that transformed the author's self-understanding

To support positive mental health:

The key issue here is to be honest with yourself about the feelings that you have and the situation you are in. This is much easier said than done! Next is the huge step of asking for help, whether from a counsellor or friend. But not all friends are up to this task, so choose wisely. A good therapist should provide a 'safe haven' so that you can feel confident to explore what's troubling you. You also have a responsibility to yourself—including the need to be open and to think realistically—so don't forget self-therapy, which can take a variety of forms.

The exercises at the back of this book will help you get started on this.

Finally, if you are able to identify your attachment status, in respect of either of your parents or carers, then that will help to give you a starting point, a base from which you can begin to make sense of your life.

Chapter 5 ~ Emerging Passions

1987–2007

1. The Blackboard Jungle

Spring term, 1987

It's the moment I've been dreading—my first day at my new, secular, state school—; how on earth will I cope? Mr Milburn, the deputy head, introduces me as a new member of staff to Year 9 in their morning assembly. He asks me to stand up, which I do, sheepishly. All Year 9 turn around to gawp at me and laugh, while I turn bright pink. Mr Milburn asks them to settle down, which they eventually do. As the assembly proceeds, I am left wondering why they laughed.

It didn't help being introduced as their new RE teacher.

Perhaps I should have worn a suit and tie instead of a jumper.

Perhaps it's because I'm rather skinny with long hair.

Perhaps it's because I looked sheepish, lacking in both confidence and authority.

Almost certainly, it's my facial expression and bodily demeanour that drew the laughter. I can tell that Year 9 are already relishing what they might get away with in RE. I can see it on their smirking faces as they leave the assembly. This is *not* where I want to be! But it's a job.

*

Fortunately, it's Monday, my lightest teaching day, with four free periods in which to contemplate my fate. It's only a few weeks since Francesca left me and I've just started therapy with Maggie. My private life is such a mess! I'm feeling very bleak, and that's *before* I meet Year 9!

One positive difference from my previous school is that I'm not responsible in any way for taking assemblies. Thank God for that! I can just stick to teaching. However, having to teach RE is a problem in itself. I'm not trained for anything else, but I'd rather teach anything else than RE! I want to ditch *all* religion in whatever shape or form and having to teach RE—and trying to make it look interesting—seems like a Herculean task, and I'm no Hercules! Neither is there any 6th form work: just four average-ability students in Year 11 studying Sikhism for 'O' level. So I'll need to mug *that* up! Then no more exam classes coming through. That's it. It's very depressing.

To make matters worse, RE has no status in the school. There are no internal exams, no fixed syllabus and no committed teachers for the past few years. Not even a head of department! It's a non-subject, yet some poor fool has to do it. So now I'm IT—the only RE teacher in a big school! Yet the Head expects me to set and mark homework every week for all of the 24 lower school classes! There isn't even a proper RE room, so I'm teaching all over the place—including art rooms, science labs and domestic science rooms. Two staff members offer me some space on their classroom display-boards, which I appreciate. They probably feel sorry for me, but not half as sorry as I feel for myself.

*

Most of my Year 7 classes are okay. One or two naughty kids, but you expect that and I handle these classes reasonably well. Even a bit of enthusiasm from some, although not generated by me, I can assure you. When I set them homework, I get about 20 out of 30 returns. The other 10 go into detention—but it's very laborious, both marking homework and checking who's attended detention—then chasing up those who haven't. So I cut a few corners: I set short 'homeworks' and allow them to do it in class time! It's still got to be marked—but this way I might cope.

Year 8 is where the trouble starts, with noisier classes and more bolshy kids: "Why do we have to do RE? It's so boring!" is a familiar cry.

I *want* to say "I totally agree with you!" but of course, I can't. I promise to try to make it more interesting. But how? As the senior staff don't seem bothered about RE, I ditch as much of the traditional stuff as I can. Instead, I introduce a more humanistic and moral approach, producing questionnaires for the pupils to answer and then discuss together in class. Questions like: *Why is there something rather than nothing? How do you tell right from wrong?* and *Is there a heaven and hell?* This approach proves far more successful than the legacy I had inherited, but I keep it quiet from senior staff until, that is, the Head calls me into his office one day.

"Mr Adams, I've had a complaint from some of our cleaning staff. They tell me there are left-wing wing posters appearing in rooms where you teach RE. Is this correct?"

"I've asked the pupils to make posters on any of the topics we'd been discussing in class. There are a couple of *Greenpeace* posters and a *Ban the Bomb* poster, among many others, which the children see as moral issues. It was completely their own choice."

"That seems perfectly reasonable to me. I'll take a look for myself at lunchtime. So off you go—and keep up the good work!"

I leave the Head's study in a bit of a daze. I think I've just earned my first brownie point!

My daze doesn't last long however—Year 9 are waiting for me!

*

Year 9 are the worst of the Year groups. A lot of background disruption and some outright bad behaviour. I struggle for control and am driven to breaking point at times. Mr Milburn tells me that I can send any trouble-makers directly to his office and this is a great help—except he won't want to see a whole class lined up against his wall! As bad luck would have it, I get most Year 9 classes towards the end of the week, with the worst two classes on Friday afternoon. Even before the afternoon starts, I'm tense and anxious and wound up like a spring. On one occasion, pupil x, who's cheeky and continually backchats me, goads me too much. I try to remove him from the room, but he thinks he can run away or hide under his desk to amuse the rest of the class. But I am far from amused! He underestimates me, as I walk right into his desk and knock it, and the chair, and pupil x, flying. It's completely unprofessional and a teacher would be reprimanded for it today. But I can hear a pin drop as the class buffoon dusts himself down and limps out of the classroom towards Mr Milburn's office. My knee is hurting, but there's no way I'm going to show it. The pupils are clearly shocked, and that particular class never troubles me again, including pupil x.

On another occasion, a full-blown fight breaks out between two boys as I'm writing on the blackboard. They are big lads for Year 9, but there's only one thing for it. I wade in with my skinny frame and manage to separate them. One steps back, realising he's in trouble. But the other remains defiant: "Let go of my arm—else I'll fuckin' nut you." I believe him and let go of his arm, not wishing to be nutted in front of the class—or at all, for that matter. I manage to escort him to Mr Milburn, while keeping a foot of clear space around him at all times.

Later that year, another troublesome pupil suddenly comes out with a load of expletives directed at me—'pissing' this and 'fucking' that—and worse. The class is as shocked as I am, but I manage to get him out of the room, with him effing and blinding as he goes. I return visibly shocked and some of the class ask if I'm alright, which I appreciate. The next day, I go and see his form tutor who gives me some information in confidence: "Don't judge him too harshly, Jamie. Nine months ago, he saw his father commit suicide, shot himself in the head. The lad has been disturbed ever since and no wonder."

This makes me think, and from that day on, when anyone makes trouble in class, I always wonder what's going on behind the scenes. I have to exert discipline as best I can, but I try to be measured. I may be working in a blackboard jungle, but some of the pupils arrive at school each day from the darkest of threatening forests.

*

I realise that I'm never going to win over the current Year 9, so I just hope I can socialise Year 7 into RE for next year and that things will slowly improve. And they do—slowly. In September, my new timetable is more complicated, so other staff are asked to teach RE and it's my job to enthuse and support them. That's difficult when I'm not enthused myself, but I provide as much practical help as I can.

Later on that year, I'm invited to a meeting where, to my surprise, everyone else is a senior member of staff. It's to discuss the problems of delivering a 'roundabout' of social education lessons (sex, drugs and the like) to Year 11. I'm relieved that there's some clever people in the room to sort out a seemingly impossible task. That is, until the meeting ends and the Head turns to *me*: "Mr Adams, we're all very busy people so we would like *you* to sort it out and report back to us in two weeks' time. Thank you. And keep up the good work!"

Do they think I'm a general dogsbody? Or do they think I might have a brain? It's hard to tell.

Nevertheless, I make a start and, after detailed conversations with all the members of staff involved, I come up with a cunning plan—and a workable timetable for social education in Year 11. I've surprised myself and it was good to work on a project that wasn't RE. Dutifully, I report back with my master-plan with printed copies for all. They seem impressed. Then Mr Milburn speaks: "James, we know that Coventry City have been doing very well recently, because you've been telling us all about it! But we think that *you've* been playing a good game too, in difficult circumstances. Therefore, from next year, you will be the Head of RE, with a further scale point and a salary increase. Congratulations!"

For the first time in eighteen long months, I can see a clearing in the blackboard jungle.

Apart from the RE that is. I'm now the Head of RE: *Get me out of here!*

2. A Social Revolution
Autumn 1989

"Wir Wollen Raus! Wir Wollen Raus! We Want Out! We Want Out!"

The people of East Berlin want out! Out from the grip of communism. Out from their failing economy and out of their poor living conditions. Out into the freedom and affluence of their West Berlin friends, neighbours and relatives on the other side of the hated Wall. Rumours and reports of the demise of the Iron Curtain are spreading like wildfire. Trains from Hungary to Austria are no longer subjected to passport controls and local rural populations are cutting through the barbed wire border fences with impunity. The momentum is unstoppable and eventually, on 9 November 1989, the citizens of Berlin are allowed free movement through the Wall's main crossing points. It's time for wild celebrations as the Berlin Wall finally crumbles to dust. A massive social revolution has won the day! Under certain favourable conditions, the collective ideas and will of a people can overcome the most hardened of dictatorial institutions.

I see it all on TV. It's a gripping spectacle, with the whole world watching! I have a special feeling for Berlin, having been on both sides of the Wall in 1967 (2.3). I also feel a connection with people breaking out from high-security institutions, after my experience of the *McVicar* film only six months previously (4.5). In similar fashion, my own life is undergoing its own silent revolution.

*

The new head of academic studies, Mr Haigh, a smartly suited gent with a southern accent greets me in the staffroom one lunchtime. Previously, we'd only made small talk about football, apart from the meetings about the social education timetable, which I had eventually sorted out.

"Mr Adams, as you may know, I've just been promoted to a senior post, which means that I can no longer teach the whole of 'A' level sociology by myself. I need someone to help share the workload and I think that you're just the person for the job. What do you say?"

I'm completely stunned.

"Thank you very much, but I don't think that's for me—my degrees are in theology, and sixth-form teaching is way above me, especially a subject that I've never taken an exam in."

Mr Haigh persists: "I think you underestimate yourself. If I'm correct, your MA thesis was about society and religion. Your PGCE included a distinction in the sociology of education and you took a course in 'A' level sociology a few years ago at a local college. You also taught the sixth-form at your previous school to 'A' level every year—at least, that's what it says on your CV. Is that not correct?"

"Er…yes…that's correct. But that was 'A' level religious studies, not sociology."

"Okay. But if you're willing to take this on, you'll get all the support you need. I'll start you with sociology of the family, which is pretty straightforward, then build up from there next year. We'll pay for you to go on any courses that you think would help, even a university course if that fits. And the more sociology you teach, the less you'd have to teach those hooligans in Year 9!" he says with a wry smile. "What do you think?"

I tell him that I'd at least think about it and get back to him the following week.

This seems a massive step-up for me, for I know that 'A' level teaching and learning is hard. It's detailed. There's a lot of it! Students' futures will depend on it! Can I really do this? Will I be up to the job? From teaching Year 9 non-exam RE to teaching 'A' level sociology to the sixth-form is a massive leap. There must be some other member of staff who is better qualified and more capable than me to do it, so I put this to him.

"Not at all. Your background and the way you sorted out that social education timetable tells me you're the best person for the job. You've got an enquiring and analytical mind and the ability to take on something new. Once you get started, I'm sure you'll enjoy it."

With a certain trepidation, I agree to take it on; missing some of those bolshy Year 9 classes is an offer I simply can't refuse!

*

Mr Haigh is as good as his word and I start with sociology of the family. Despite thorough preparation, I'm very nervous for the first few weeks, never venturing more than a foot away from my notes. When we get to the 'dark side of the family', I notice some research by a certain John Bowlby. It's worth a few lines in the students' notes, but I think nothing more about it and we move on. In the following two years, Mr Haigh organises several sociology trips: in the school minibus around the better and worse parts of Nottingham to illustrate the wealth and poverty topic. To Granada Studios to illustrate the sociology of mass media, and to Skegness for an intensive revision weekend before the students' final exams. I'm learning fast and just about keeping pace with the students!

While at Granada Studios, Alex, a keen Beatles fan, asks me if she can touch the Beatles' actual drum-kit that's on display, despite the red cordon to keep people at a distance. Mr Haigh and the rest of the group have moved on, so I tell Alex that I'll look away, which I do. I see nothing…

"Thanks sir! That's amazing! It's the best day of my life!"

I tell her that celebrity icons are not only about the power of the mass media but also the sociology of religion for, according to Emile Durkheim (one of sociology's founding fathers): "A rock, a tree, a spring, a pebble, a piece of wood, a house—in a word, anything can become sacred" [95], including the Beatles drum-kit. When I come to teach the sociology of education, I'm shocked to discover that exam performance and university entrance is closely linked to social class: the higher your social class, the better will be your results and chances of university. That's dreadful and is something that I never learned on my PGCE course. I wonder why that was? Institutionalised social class bias perhaps?

Eventually, I get around to teaching the theories of Karl Marx. I find his views about 'false consciousness' really interesting—and not dissimilar to Freud's view of the unconscious: both appear to be universally true, yet neither can be verified in principle. They are indeed conundrums.

Of sociology's three founding fathers: Durkheim, Marx and Weber, I find the theories of Weber the most credible as he combines elements of Durkheim and Marx, while formulating his own contribution: that social groups can, in certain circumstances, bring about major social change without resorting to violent revolution [96]. It's called Social Action Theory and, as I watch the jubilant Berlin crowds joining hands on top of the Wall and embracing one another at the Brandenburg Gate, I can see Weber's "Action Theory" in action!

After spending two years under Mr Haigh's wing, he has another announcement for me: "Jamie, I've just accepted a headship in London. From now on, *you* are the Head of Sociology. I'm sure you'll make a great job of it. But you'll have to find someone else to teach with you."

Now that I'm fully committed to the subject, I'm confident about taking on the new role. And it gives me a new idea! So I'm soon in the Head's office with a suggestion, and leave with a huge smile on my face: *I'm no longer the Head of RE! I'm the Head of Religious and Social Studies!* It feels like a seismic shift as my personal revolution continues—as do Europe's social and political upheavals.

*

Throughout my two years' initiation into sociology, I've been on a number of day courses that introduce me to new topics and exam marking, and on a weekend course at York for teachers new to the subject. I also sign up for an MA in sociology at Nottingham University. I don't need another MA, but I do need more sociology under my belt. The course is very interesting—especially the evening lectures on *Health and Social Class*, *The Inner City* and *The Sociology of Everyday Life*.

I'm absorbed by *The Sociology of Everyday Life*—for there's a fascinating coherence with the Transactional Analysis I've been learning with Maggie (4.2). One Christmas holiday, I sit down and type for four hours without a single break. When I try to get up, my back is solid and there's a ringing in my ears—I've got tinnitus through short-term stress overload: the result of getting too passionate about my new academic interests! Passion is a risky business, whether at work or play!

By the end of that Christmas holiday, I'd written a 10,000-word thesis on *The Sociology of Emotion: Understanding Emotions as Social Actions.* It's been derived from the evening lectures and from two recommended books [97]. I want to connect Weber's *Social Action theory* and Goffman's *Symbolic Interactionism* with Berne's *Transactional Analysis*. It's an ambitious project that addresses concepts like *framing, emotion-work, impression-management, front-stage* and *back-stage, surface-acting* and *deep-acting, merging* and the *false-self.* It argues that emotions can be prompted and moulded by the external social world—meaning that they have external as well as internal triggers.

My MA tutor reads it and considers it a possible starting point for an M.Litt. degree. But I have other fish to fry (4.8). Back at school, my Year 11 social education students are in the process of igniting their own revolution: "*We Want Out! We Want Out!*"

So I ask them: "Out of what? And why?" (5.4)

3. Crisis in the Classroom

*If you have not yet done the Ego-gram exercise (Appendix B), then this is a good time to do it, before reading on.

It's Wednesday afternoon and it's raining outside. Inside, I have a double period of social education with Year 11 and the natives are getting restless. I'm struggling to maintain control and continue with the lesson, when Jodie shoots her hand up: "Please sir…"

I'm glad it's Jodie—she always has something constructive to say, so that will ease the pressure for a while.

"Yes Jodie?"

"I don't mean to be horrible, sir, but we all think what we're doing is *very* boring! Can't we do something else?"

I'm shocked by Jodie's negativity. I've never heard her speak like this before and judging by the sudden silence of the class, neither had they. You can cut the atmosphere with a knife as they await my answer.

I realise that I've a crisis on my hands, so I need to buy myself some time.

"Thank you, Jodie. It's nearly the end of the first lesson, so talk among yourselves for a few minutes and I'll see what I can do. And quietly please!"

Momentarily, this pacifies the natives, as I turn my back on them and wander into a corner. My lessons on 'evil and suffering' clearly aren't working—but what can I do?! I don't have a plan B—or C. I'm well and truly stuck and I fear a full-scale revolution.

Then suddenly, from nowhere, a revelation—a visual image—of a lesson at theological college from over twenty years previously. I see a blackboard and on the blackboard, there is the outline of an iceberg with sea level nine-tenths of the way up. There are five words written on this diagram: *conscious*; *unconscious*; *id; ego; superego*. I realise that it's Freud's 'iceberg diagram' of the human mind. I've got nothing else so let's give it a go.

*

I draw the diagram on the blackboard, exactly as I see it in my mind. I then walk around the room and place a blank sheet of paper on every student's desk. I return to the front, turn, face the class and wait for silence.

"Okay folks, listen up! Here's what we're going to do. First, copy down the diagram on the blackboard, including the words, even though you won't understand some of them."

They get busy copying, while I breathe a sigh of relief. So far, so good.

"When you've finished the diagram, look up and I'll explain *id*. Then, in pairs, think of some examples and write them down. You've got three minutes. We'll do *superego* next."

It seems to be going quite well. I'm waiting for trouble—but I don't get any. As they give their examples, we discuss them. I explain the conflict between the id and the superego—and they give examples of that too. Same with the conscious and the unconscious—we discuss it all. Before we know it, the bell sounds and the crisis is over!

As the students are leaving, Jodie and her friends come over.

"That was really interesting, sir, can we do some more next week?"

"Sorry Jodie, that's your last week with me. It's drugs with Miss Smith next week! But thanks for speaking up today—you did the right thing."

After that, I drop my four-week course on 'evil and suffering' and work out how I can use the iceberg lesson—but over four weeks. It dawns on me that Freud's id, ego and superego correspond to the Child, Adult and Parent of Transactional Analysis. I could do an introduction to TA using the iceberg diagram—to get the students thinking psychologically; then a lesson with the Ego-gram; a lesson on the various types of transactions; and a final lesson for them to role-play these, to learn how to improve communication (4.2). It's worth a try so I start to prepare materials for my new social education topic.

*

After teaching my new TA course once, I'm 100% convinced that I'm doing the right thing. The students are more engaged and less challenging than previously, and I also notice something else. At the end of most lessons, a few students come to thank me and say a cheery goodbye. At the end of the final session, several ask me if they can do some more the following week, which they can't as it's only a four-week course. This isn't a one-off incident—it happens more times than not. Something seems to be connecting.

I also notice that, in the second week, when various students ask me to interpret their ego-grams, they are shocked by how well I seem to know them just by looking at five shaded-in bar charts on a bit of paper! Some think I'm a mind reader, which I assure them I'm not! The following year, the Head of English tells me that some of her 'A' level literature group have been using the concepts of TA that they had learnt the previous year to analyse various characters in Shakespeare's plays. She's very impressed and so am I.

Word is getting around about my TA course and within a year or so, four members of staff, including senior staff, attend TA courses so that it can be delivered to Year 9 social education classes as well [98]. Obviously, for me it's very gratifying but I'm not at all prepared for what happens next: "*We want out! We want out!*"

A group of Year 11 students stand before me at the end of their four-week TA course. They are not poorly behaved or difficult students. To the contrary, they're some of the best and brightest students in the school. So what's going on?

"We don't want to stay at this school. We all want to go to a sixth-form college instead, unless…"

"Unless what?" I ask.

It's another crisis in the classroom.

4. Student Power

"Unless YOU can teach us 'A' level psychology! We'd rather stay here with our friends but we all want to do 'A' level psychology—and it's not offered here. So we're hoping that you could introduce it. Otherwise, we want to be out of here and off to a sixth-form college. So, can you teach it? If you can, we'll get up a petition to the Head."

I'm lost for words but fortunately, it's morning break and I've a free period next, so I can chat with them for a few minutes and gather my thoughts. I'd overheard in the staffroom about a 'brain-drain' from the current Year 11 to the local sixth-form college. So it seems that I'm at the sharp end! Fortunately, I've been reading a lot of psychology over the past year. Not only TA and Attachment Theory, but the mainstream theories: psychodynamic, biological, behaviourist and cognitive. I've delved into developmental psychology, abnormal psychology, Sigmund Freud, John Bowlby and Carl Rogers. It's a bit of a mixed bag—but I've developed a passion for the subject.

By the end of break, I've had time to think and I give them my considered reply: "Yes, I think it's possible, and I'd love to do it. But there are a few provisos:

1. I need to see an 'A' level syllabus first—several, if possible.
2. I can't teach it all, so I'd need someone else to teach it with me.
3. I want to see your petition before you take it to the Head.

"So come back next week and we'll see where we're at. Okay?"

"Thanks sir! That's brilliant! We'll start getting some signatures!"

I'm both surprised and flattered by their confidence in me. But it may be just a flash in the-pan and that by next week, they'll all be wanting to do politics, law or Greek philosophy! We'll see.

The following week they all turn up, petition in hand, still enthused about 'A' level psychology in the sixth form. There's twenty signatures, all of them bright, capable and hard-working students. I suggest they tone down the wording from 'demand' to 'request'—then off they go with their petition to Mr Milburn, who has recently been promoted to Head Teacher.

*

Ten days later, he calls me into his office to discuss the petition (4.9). He's clearly concerned to stem the 'brain-drain' from the sixth-form and agrees, in principle, to my introducing 'A' level psychology in the next academic year. Furthermore, he has some good news to tell me.

"I've recently received a letter from a retired psychology teacher and examiner who's just moved into the area. He's looking for part-time work. Obviously, I need to see him first but he could be ideal. He could teach the parts of the syllabus that you don't feel able to and I'd give you an extra free period a week so that he could tutor you. The school will give you £500 to set up the department with books and other materials. So if everything works out, you'll be Head of Psychology as well as Sociology and RS. Good luck!"

As it turns out, the retired Mr Filbert knows his psychology inside out and is more than happy to teach the more scientific parts of the syllabus that I can't get my head around. His weekly tutoring is excellent, especially on those topics that are new to me.

The first group of students—those who had organised the petition—are a dream to teach. Mr Filbert and I are also impressed by the way the students revise together—even around each other's houses, especially as their first exam in 'AS Psychology' approaches. When Results Day arrives in August, we are all very nervous. But the nerves soon disappear when we see the results: all students have passed and half the group have achieved 'A' grades! Of those, two students have achieved 100%—something that Mr Filbert has rarely seen before as an examiner. Our joint efforts, and the students' collaborative work and thorough revision, have won the day!

From then on, in the following years, 'A' level psychology starts to attract increasing numbers of students, which they often combine with sociology. It's difficult to take it all in as, thanks to student power, the RSS department goes from strength to strength—and I am teaching less and less RS! However, at the same time that school is going so well for me, my social life is rapidly turning into a disaster zone!

5. Single and Mingling

Mike is not his usual buoyant self and I'm wondering why, but he soon spits it out: *"Jamie, I've some bad news for you, although it's really good news for me. I've been accepted as the Senior Lecturer in Politics at the University of Melbourne, and I'm leaving in two months."*

This is a severe blow. I know he had been looking for a new challenge, but I had thought he was only looking in the UK. Naturally, I'm happy for him, but it puts me in a quandary; for since my relationship with Karla, Mike has been my main source of social life. Of course, I've continued to date women, occasionally with success. But I've not found any connection or any real passion in the dating game. I've not needed it so much because Mike has always been an excellent friend, whether going to football, playing pool, discussing politics or even reviewing my latest date. We'd also holidayed together on several occasions. He's excellent company. Now that he's going, what's to become of my social life?

*

As Mike heads for sunnier climes, I need to take action, but I can't simply do more dating. I need something different.

I start by joining *Spice*, an organisation for thirty-somethings and beyond, who enjoy a bit of a challenge. I attend a basic pub night—a challenge in itself for me as I'm not a drinker. No one makes any effort to speak to me and I find it hard to talk to people I don't know. Perhaps they think I'm a bit old for them. They seem a bit cliquey. But I sign up for some tennis as I like competitive sports. All goes well at the tennis evening as I get stuck into a game with an equally matched partner when the evening's organiser suddenly switches us around— and now I'm playing doubles with a mixed bag of abilities. We're then switched again, and again—and I return home disappointed. Never mind, football is more my game, so I'll try some 5-a-side soccer. Again, everything is going well and

I've even scored a goal to give us a 2-1 lead, when the ref—who is the *Spice* organiser—awards our opponents a penalty on the grounds that the game needs to be evened up a bit! So it's now 2-2. We manage to score again—but the same happens. A game of football that no one can win! It's a joke! And that was the end of *Spice* for me. I didn't fancy bungee-jumping anyway.

*

My next move is to join *Nexus*, specifically a club for single people, and more my age group. Again, I start with a basic pub night, which goes okay, until I return to find that my car has been stolen! So that's a bit of a downer, but I'm not put off. I try out some *Nexus* activities: I go on a couple of walks, I attend a barbeque or two and I turn up at a dance evening. But once again, I find that all my conversations are superficial. Even if you start to have a really good chat with someone, they are always liable to suddenly break off with: "I'm sorry, but I need to mingle!" Perhaps it's me. Perhaps no one is interested in Coventry City's 1987 Cup Final success, or in Transactional Analysis, or Attachment theory. I can't think why—they're the three most interesting things on the planet! So I'm getting pretty depressed with all my unsuccessful efforts to establish a social life.

Except, that is, for one thing. When I was at the dance evening, although I could only jig about rather pathetically, I did notice something else: the smell of alcohol (though I don't drink), the stink of cigarettes (though I don't smoke) and the seduction of ladies' perfume (though I do pull if given half a chance): when combined, I find them enchanting! Especially when I'm around those ladies who are still very attractive in their forties and know it, and who are happy to reveal some flesh. So I come to realise that I love the whiff of decadence! Be it in a pub, a nightclub or a dance hall.

*

With this in mind, I take myself off to a *Nexus* Christmas Eve dinner-dance in a large Grantham hotel. It's attended by other people with works parties and the like—*Nexus* has just one table. After the meal is finished and the tables cleared, the lights are dimmed and the dancing starts. I stand by a pillar, admiring those who can dance, trying to look nonchalant, orange juice in hand. Then, out of the shadows appears a very attractive young lady, tall, slim and dusky with jet-black hair in ringlets. She's gorgeous and she's heading for me!

After brief introductions, Maria leads me onto the dance floor for a slow dance with her arms locked around my neck. Has Santa come early? Will her stockings be on my floor in the morning? I'm aware of the whiskey glass she's holding behind my head, so perhaps she's drunk and that's why she's hit on me. We enjoy a smoochy dance or two, and my interest is beginning to rise—when she starts asking me a few questions: "So, my darling, what's your line of work? And what sort of car do you drive?"

Foolishly, I tell the truth: "I'm a sociology teacher and I drive an Astra."

Within a few minutes, she's off to 'powder her nose'—and that's the last I see of her. It's only later that I realise that I should have powdered my reply with a few white lies. She wasn't interested in pulling a sociology teacher who drives an Astra. She wants a minted solicitor who drives an Audi! I console myself with the thought that I was initially fanciable, together with some *what if* fantasies.

My next *Nexus* dance is at the end of January. I'm becoming more and more envious of the couples on the dance floor who are doing rock 'n' roll, jive, salsa or tango. I want to be on the dance floor too, rather than on the edge, looking on. I notice a young lady also on the edge and looking on, someone who I've seen at previous *Nexus* events but to whom I've never spoken. Eventually, we get chatting, and we're still chatting after everyone else has left. We exchange phone numbers and before long, we're chatting in bed at hers, then a week later at mine. For the first time in several years, I receive a Valentine's Day card, and I take her out for a Valentine's Day meal. Beth can be a bit sharp with her tongue, but she's good fun in between the sheets.

A few weeks later, I suggest over the phone that we might go away together over Easter. Beth seems up for this, until I suggest that we each pay our own way.

"You can forget that! Bugger off!" came her less-than-cultured reply.

"So you've never heard of women's equality?" is my riposte. She clearly hasn't as she puts the phone down even before I finish speaking. And that was that with Beth. Well—almost.

As fate would have it, the very next day there is a *Nexus* 'Vicars, Tarts and Tramps' evening house-party, to which I intend to go as it sounds interestingly decadent. It is. The music gets going quickly and there's very little small talk, with people drinking and dancing nonstop until midnight. There's no couples dancing as there's not much room, so I'm happy jigging about with everyone else.

I notice that Beth is here, but we make no effort to talk to each other. I'm assuming that I got dumped over the phone the previous night. As it happens, Cassie seems to be taking a fancy to me, so I decide to take a fancy to her, especially as Beth is jigging around next to us, giving me the evil eye. I seize the opportunity for a bit of couples-dancing with Cassie, and we slow-dance very intimately with each other. As our entwined bodies slowly rotate, I see Beth at every rotation giving me the 'evils'—which I much enjoy. *What goes around, comes around*, I think to myself. After all, it was she who dumped me—I'm just letting her know that I'm happy to be dumped.

Ten days later, I'm around Cassie's house, making love in front of her log-fire. A week after that, we're trying out a sheepskin rug at my place. Thereafter, neither of us makes contact again. We're just not that interested—but it was fun for a few weeks.

*

In search of further decadence, I start to attend a Singles dance every Sunday evening in a large Nottingham hotel. After three weeks, I'm starting to recognise a few faces, even though I don't do much dancing and I'm pretty useless at chatting women up. Women seem more defensive here than they do at *Nexus* dances—but those dances are only once a month. On the balance of probability, I feel sure that my luck will change and that a Maria or a Cassie or someone else will hit on me. So I keep going, especially as the music is always good.

However, on one memorable occasion, things are particularly bad. When I ask ladies for a dance, I don't get rejected just a few times. I get rejected *every time*—nine times before I eventually leave. They don't even say 'No thank you'. They just turn their backs on me and close ranks. I'm devastated. Perhaps after all, neither dancing nor decadence is for me. I scuttle back home in the dark, vowing never to go there again. The familiar whiff of isolation and emptiness swirls around me and within. How I long for school, for sociology and psychology lessons and my sixth-form students!

As for my social life, I'm still very single and struggling to mingle.

6. Love and Lust
(On the Dance Floor)
Summer 1996

"Jamie, you should see the women that go there!
They are very nice—and lots of them!"

I suddenly perk up after a long evening of superficial chat at a *Nexus* pub-night. Paul has just arrived, late as usual. I can talk to him—he's a Nottingham Forest supporter, so we often talk football. On this occasion, we discuss my recent bad experience at the Singles dance night in Nottingham, and how I really want to dance properly.

"You should go to St John's church hall on a Monday night. It's called *Ceroc*. It doesn't seem too difficult to me, and I've got two left feet! The women are really nice!"

*

I make an excuse not to go the following Monday as I'm cautious about being plunged in at the deep end. I might have two left feet as well! The thought of meeting lots of new people is also daunting, and there's *Monday Night Football* on *Sky*. So I flunk it. By the following Monday, curiosity has got the better of me and I'm bang on time at the church hall. Paul's there—and he's right about the women too. The dance teacher also catches my eye: wow! Attractive, tall and leggy, with the shortest of short dance-skirts.

Suddenly, I'm grabbed by the hand by a middle-aged lady who I recognise from *Nexus*. She leads me to the line, as the class gets going. I'm still ogling the dance teacher so I mishear an instruction and make a mistake. My partner helps me sort it out, but I repeat the mistake—I just don't get it. The women then move on to new partners so now I'm with someone else. It starts to get more complicated as we begin a second move and I'm asked to cross my right hand over the left, turn the lady clockwise and then step back. Information overload! Which is my right hand? *That* one! Which is my left hand? It must be *this* one! Now which one goes over which? I'm confused!

I look up from my hands to yet another new lady in front of me and I see my previous partner giving me a funny look as she moves down the line. Everyone else seems to be getting it, apart from me! I fumble the next move too. It's all too much, so I drop out of the line. I didn't expect it to be *this* difficult! I'm totally uncoordinated. Maybe I've been living in my head so much, with all these -ologies, that I've no physical awareness of my body parts. Apart from one.

I'm frustrated, upset and angry. I'll never get this! I'll never be a dancer! I walk out, bashing open the internal swing doors as I make a dramatic exit. Let me get back to the safe familiarity of *Coronation Street* or the second half of the football.

*

Outside, it's still light and the sky is clear. My head starts to clear too. I think about the lovely young ladies inside the hall. And the dance teacher! So why am I going home just to watch TV? Suddenly, a TA thought springs to mind. Aren't I being rather Child-ish? Can I not step into my Adult, go back inside the hall and have another go? Then, if that fails, perhaps I'm just not cut out for dancing. That sounds a better idea than simply giving up at the first hurdle.

I return inside, watch the other dancers carefully and then wait for the next class to start. This is the intermediate class, so I'm expecting it to be harder. But now that I've got my left and right hands sorted out, it's not too bad. With a bit more concentration and with help from my various partners, I manage the first two moves, and then make progress with the third and fourth. When it's finished, I'm pretty pleased with myself and make for the bar.

I'm drinking alone when the freestyle starts—when people can practise the moves they've just learnt and more experienced dancers can dance how they wish. I want to have another go, but I don't know anyone apart from Paul and I don't want to dance with him, nice guy though he is. At the table next to me, there are four attractive young ladies chatting away to each other. I pluck up as much courage as I can muster and go over. They all look up. I feel very exposed, but blurt out: "I'm Jamie. I'm a beginner and probably a hopeless case—but could any of you help me out?"

There's a pregnant pause, before one speaks up: "Jamie, I'll be delighted to help you. I'm Davinia. Come on. Let's start with the Arm-jive."

Davinia is totally gorgeous in every sense of the word. I guess she's about thirty, polite and well-spoken, with a neat, trim figure and a lovely smile. She explains things clearly and doesn't rush me.

She suggests I get a bit closer to her, hip-to-hip. It's pretty scary feeling her body so close to mine—but I do my best! After twenty minutes, she suggests I dance with one of her friends, which I do, and then come back to her later. Eventually, I have to sit down for a minute as I try to absorb the evening. But not for long, as I get an unexpected invitation from…the dance teacher!

"Come on, Jamie, show me what you can do!" she says, teasing me with a smile. She pulls me up and I try out the moves I think I've learnt.

"Come closer, come closer! Don't dance so far away!" She pulls me in closer so that I feel every contour of her body. She's super-confident, while I'm a quivering wreck! But I like it—her body, that is! Finally, I return to Davinia and ask her for the last dance of the evening.

"I'll be delighted to dance with you, Jamie!" Words I have never forgotten. Davinia, my first dance partner, was always 'delighted' to dance with me— before moving away to London six months later. She made a big impression on me about how to treat beginners: "We were all beginners once", which challenged me about how sympathetically I treated struggling pupils at school.

*

From that first dramatic evening, I'm hooked on *Ceroc*. There are sixteen basic moves and we learn four every week in the beginner's class. Within a month, I'm a reasonably competent dancer. Having two left feet or not doesn't matter as it's a hand-led dance with virtually no footwork to learn. The music is popular and upbeat and the dance ethic is democratic: you dance with anyone who asks, and anyone you ask will also dance with you. Women ask men to dance just as men ask women. It's sociable! It's sexy! It's great! There's just one snag. Well, two actually.

The first is that male-female relationships seem very different from the outside world. For example, if you enjoy eye contact, as I do, it's very difficult to know what is meant when it's reciprocated. I enjoy warm, flirtatious eye contact with many of the ladies, only to discover that they are wearing a wedding ring! I'm delighted with the close bodily contact that some young women thrust on me, slipping their legs in between mine, but then there's nothing after that. Are they just teasing me for the fun of it, or what? When is someone coming on to me and when are they just enjoying dancing close? It's a minefield for misunderstanding, and after forty classes and freestyle dances in six months, I am no nearer to finding a girlfriend—or even a dance partner.

The second snag is that *Ceroc* is frenetic, with frequent partner changes, so there's little opportunity to talk, apart from superficial snatches of conversation while you're dancing. Even if I start a conversation while watching the dancing or having a drink, either myself or my companion can be whisked onto the dance floor at any moment. Yes—it's a hundred times better than a *Nexus* pub night— but conversation rarely gets beyond the superficial.

*

About nine months after I start dancing, one of the best female dancers at St John's asks me, much to my surprise, if we can go together to the Singles dance night in Nottingham—the one where I had experienced such a bad time before I started *Ceroc*. I'm cautious but as we shall go as a couple; I'm ready to give it a try. Maisie is a pleasant young lady with a trim figure and I'm also keen to go Ceroc-dancing whenever I can.

During the car ride over, I discover that Maisie is a lecturer in philosophy at Nottingham—I'm impressed! Especially as her specialist subject is Postmodernism, which I'm currently teaching to my 'A' level sociology students as a new perspective about society. Before we reach our dance venue, we've already discussed the end of 'Grand Narratives', the dominance of image over reality and that 'nothing is solid' in our ever-changing world and consciousness. For me, it's a great start to the evening.

As the Singles night clientele don't start dancing till later, we have the whole dance floor to ourselves and we turn a few heads as we jive and spin in unison, up and down the ballroom. Maisie is a great dancer and I feel that I'm keeping up reasonably well. I really hope that all those 'Singles' who had rejected me so recently are watching me now!

As the floor eventually fills up, we have less room to ourselves and Maisie asks me if I know any *seducers*. I'm tempted to make a quip, but I allow her to explain these more advanced moves. She shows me how to lower her down for a first-move drop, a ballroom drop and a lambada. It's very intimate! So we practise a few of them before our last dance, and then we call it a night.

After a great evening, we head back to Grantham and she invites herself in for coffee at my place. It's getting late and I've a psychology lesson to finish preparing, for first thing in the morning. When I return with the coffee, I'm expecting to find her browsing my bookshelves for my Postmodern paperbacks. Instead, I find her stretched out on the sofa, with her dance shoes kicked off and looking decidedly dishevelled. She beckons me to join her and I do so without hesitation, having already decided that my psychology lesson is prepared enough. With coffee half-drunk, I ask her if she'd like to move upstairs.

"I thought you'd never ask!" as she takes my hand and leads the way.

*

We enjoy the next two Sundays in similar fashion: dancing, decadence and Derrida—a postmodern writer. It's a heady mix and Maisie is definitely growing on me. That's a pity for at the next local dance, I'm looking out for her—but she waltzes in with a new man in tow and cuts me dead with a single glance.

Nothing is solid! I smile to myself in a form of gallows humour. *Everything is in flux.*

I quickly realise that it was only lust and not love and, to be sure, a bit of postmodern lusting was fun—but for me, it's not enough. I'm wanting something more from the dance floor and before too long, that's exactly what I get.

7. Too Much

It's several months later when I meet Georgie—not on the dance floor but at school. She's doing some temporary supply work for a member of staff who's off sick. As a couple of those lessons are for RE, for which I am responsible, I need to induct her into the Year 8 scheme of work. Over a sandwich and soup lunch, we have time to chat, during which she pours out her troubles about a never-ending legal settlement concerning her divorce and business venture with her ex. She seems a bit fragile and it's in everyone's interests, not least her own, that she continues to work. As I'm free for one of her two RE periods, I support her as much as I can in the classroom.

*

Then, at the end of her first week, she asks me if I'd like to go to a live gig with her at a Nottingham Soul & Blues club—as live music is her thing. I accept her offer and we go in her car. Inside the club, it's dark, loud and sweaty but pleasantly decadent! Eventually, some folks take to the floor and so do we; although it's not exactly *Ceroc*! On the rough timber that passes for a dance floor, Georgie cuts a fine figure as she dances—slim, petite and curvy with a long ponytail.

Back at her place just after midnight, I'm curious to find out more about her lifestyle. But hardly before I'm in the door, she's propelling me against the wall and unzipping my leather jacket. With her hands inside the jacket, she leans up to kiss me, long and deep, until I feel I'm being swallowed whole! I've never been kissed with such open-mouthed passion before! Especially on a first date! And it leaves me wondering…but not for long as she's soon taking me upstairs. It's the start of something new and I'm not complaining—for at last, it seems, I've met a lady who's really into me and who doesn't seem likely to reject me. As our relationship progresses, I take her to a *Ceroc* dance but she quickly decides that it's not her scene. In particular, she doesn't like me dancing with other women—she wants me all to herself. So we spend most Friday and Saturday evenings at her choice of live music venues, but when we occasionally try *Ceroc* for a change, then she's not a happy bunny and we don't stay for long. So there's often a bit of underlying tension on our nights out. She seems completely devoted to me, which is something I'm enjoying, but I'm totally not used to.

*

Apart from her dislike of *Ceroc*, things are going well with Georgie. She can't do enough for me: in small, practical ways, as well as in bed. She's eager, pretty and very sensual—a thoroughly modern young woman, who is confident to lead the way in the bedroom. We continue to have endless discussions about her legal problems and divorce—and these huge burdens start to loom large in an otherwise happy relationship. I'm quite a good listener and I want to help her as much as I can. But I'm starting to feel under-whelmed by her live music and overwhelmed by her loving, and I'm finding this a difficult balancing act.

But isn't this what I've been wanting all these years? A girlfriend who is totally into me, with not a single doubt about her leaving? I should be the happiest man in the world. But I'm not.

*

As the months turn into a year, I'm starting to have doubts, though I'm not sure why—so I ignore them for as long as I can. Things come to a head one Sunday morning. After our usual frisky nights, we usually wake up to enjoy long sensuous mornings in bed. But on this particular morning, I *feel* nothing. Thinking Georgie is still asleep and knowing that *Match of the Day*—the Sunday morning repeat—is about to start, I creep downstairs, eager to catch up on my missed football. But my escape doesn't last long; Georgie is standing at the doorway in a short, black negligee, and declares me to be seriously offside. Like a naughty boy, I return upstairs to the field of satin sheets, where I realise with a shock that I really am more interested in the football, although I really wish I wasn't. So, this morning, there's still plenty of loving touches but no actual love-making. My body just isn't interested, however much I'd like it to be. And I've no idea why.

The same situation—my lack of desire—repeats itself in the following weeks and I have to admit to myself, though not yet to Georgie, that my feelings for her are changing. I phone Katie—a long-standing dance friend who knows me well—for a chat. Katie always has something wise and sensible to say about relationships—she's had a few herself, though not with me. She eventually expresses her own thoughts about Georgie and myself: "Jamie, you seem to spend a lot of time listening to Georgie's problems, but how often does she listen to yours? You also seem to have given up Coventry City recently. It seems a rather one-sided relationship to me."

"Never mind about that; what about the sex stuff? I want to make love but I can't. She's a gorgeous, delicious, young lady, but I'm just not hungry for her! I should be in seventh heaven. But I'm not."

Katie tells me that these issues are above her pay-grade and suggests I talk to Maggie, my long-term counsellor, which I do.

Maggie suggests that Georgie and myself are both very needy people—albeit for different reasons—and that this is not a good basis for a relationship.

"Forget the relationship stuff, what about the sex?" I plead.

Maggie pauses a second. "I suspect that in your case, the relationship and the sex are very much related. I think it's about Georgie's *availability.* Sexually, you seem more excited by unconventional or precarious relationships, where your girlfriends are unpredictable or, as in Francesca's case, still married. In other words, they are not fully available. This unstable dynamic is what you're used to—starting with your inconsistently available mother. Georgie is the first lady you've mentioned who is completely available to you, apart from Sophie, that is. And with Sophie, when sex was *unavailable* before you got engaged, you were super-keen. But when she became sexually available once you became engaged, your interest waned, then died. Is this not true?"

I leave Maggie's house with explosive thoughts going off in my head, as on my earlier visits. I don't like the logic of her suggestion or the implications it has, not only for me and Georgie, but for any future relationship of mine as well. So I decide to label it: 'just a suggestion', along with our mutual neediness, as another possible factor for my loss of desire. I console myself with the thought that "it's complicated" and leave it at that.

But sex, or rather the lack of it, remains a problem. We're both continually disappointed so eventually, I decide to break it off. She's very upset, although we continue to meet and talk, which seems to smooth things over. It also helps that, by now, she's doing supply work at another school.

It's clear that we're both lonely and that we are still drawn to each other. Therefore, as a compromise arrangement, we arrange to meet for dates once a month—and invariably end up in bed together. Georgie continues to overwhelm me with her affection and I continue to under-perform, although we both enjoy the skin-to-skin contact. But each time, I return home the following morning, having spent the night with Georgie and I'm glad that I'm free to be myself again for another month. To me it's a good arrangement: *we're friends with benefits*, I tell myself, and I assume that it's the same for Georgie—but of course, it's not. For Georgie needs far more benefits than I am able to offer.

We continue our monthly dates as we try to give love a second and even a third chance. We both want the relationship to work, but that's not enough to overcome the emotional baggage that we are both contributing to the relationship. Therefore, eventually and reluctantly, I bring it to a permanent conclusion—leaving Georgie bitterly disappointed and by now very angry with me for having raised and dashed her hopes so many times.

I'm also feeling angry and upset—not with Georgie, but with myself and my physical inability to respond to her in the way that we both wanted. I'm also confused about why I'm rejecting such affection and love when it's handed to me on a plate! And then, I remember her very first kiss and realise how it has both symbolised and prefigured our whole relationship! I didn't want to be swallowed whole then, or now.

With Maisie, lust was *not enough*. But with Georgie, her needy, overwhelming love was just *too much*. Which leaves me with the obvious existential question: will I ever find a love that's *just right*?

8. The Great Pretender
1999

With her sultry looks, high heels and sharp designer outfit, Amber doesn't look like your average secondary school teacher. She isn't. In fact, she's a drugs expert and is about to make a presentation at a one-day course about social education in secondary schools. She's friendly enough as we chat over coffee at the start of the day. Amber asks me what aspect of social education I'm involved with at my school.

"Transactional Analysis!" I gleefully announce, before describing its successful introduction at my school with both students and staff (5.3). She seems intrigued as she glances at her watch.

"James, I'd love to know more but I must go and set up," and off she goes.

At the end of her presentation, I manage to catch her as she's leaving and slip her my email address with 'TA' written next to it in large letters. Not for a moment do I think I will hear from her...but I do.

So I start to fantasise again about the possibility of a Miss Right or, at least, a Miss Almost Right.

*

We meet up in a city centre wine bar in Nottingham, and I immediately find six coasters and arrange them in two vertical sets of three, side by side (4.2 diagram) and start to explain the basics. I also give her an ego-gram to complete (Appendix B), which she does in the stated two minutes, once I've explained how to complete it. She seems impressed by the way I can correctly 'read' aspects of her personality from her results, especially the strong 'adaptive child' result that appears in the far right-hand column.

"Oh yes, that's me! I love dressing up and pretending to be someone else. I do amateur dramatics in my spare time—it's great!"

I ask her whether she thinks that TA might have any bearing upon her drugs expertise…

"It's hard to say but it does help explain why my boyfriend and I split up."

We continue to chat about all manner of things, including *Ceroc* dancing, which she has heard of but never tried. After an hour and a half of nonstop chat, it's time to part; as we exit the bar, she pulls me in for a hug. With her arm hooked around my neck, she kisses me on the lips. It's not a snog but it's not a peck either.

"James, I've really enjoyed talking to you. I'd like to do this again some time. I'll email you."

Then she's off, but not before she's turned around and called out: "And next time we meet, you can teach me to dance!"

*

Motionless outside the bar, I watch Amber strut off and turn the corner. I'm stunned—I hadn't seen that coming, although I had noticed and enjoyed her warm, direct eye contact as we chatted together. For the next week, I daydream about being with Amber on the dance floor, with me leading her into my favourite moves of seducers, the lambada and the comb. I imagine our first proper kiss, and where that might lead…

In the following months, we meet every week to chat and I take her to the weekly dance classes in Nottingham. We don't join in the beginners' lines, as she insists that we practise together and not with any others. She's always warm, charming and affectionate and hugs me in public without any hint of embarrassment. I'm on a high and lapping it all up.

After several carefree weeks, out of the blue, she cancels our dance class meeting for no obvious reason, which leaves me very unhappy and disappointed. Our burgeoning friendship suddenly starts to feel a bit shaky rather than solid. She then asks to meet me at a different time and place from usual and I'm soon feeling gripped with anxiety.

When we meet, I can see that Amber has a different face on, and a different tone of voice: "Jamie, I'm really sorry but I can't meet you anymore—I'm pregnant!"

I'm totally stunned by her news, not least because I know for a fact that I'm not the father! Chance would be a fine thing! Yes, I could imagine myself living with Amber and a cute little baby. Perhaps.

I feel I'm owed an explanation and I get one.

"You see, my ex-boyfriend I was telling you about decided he wanted me back. So we got back together—and now I'm pregnant! We're going to get married in the summer."

It's a lot for me to take in. I feel that I've lost her attention, her dancing and her friendship, all in one go. I have a deep sense of having been given the run-around, even of being used—although I'm not sure why. I just can't think straight.

Thankfully, my dance friend Katie has a few ideas as we discuss the recent turn of events. We come to the conclusion that Amber's initial reason for striking up a friendship with me was genuine enough. Then, realising that our friendship might make her ex-boyfriend jealous, she may have fed him information about our chats and our dancing, which had the desired effect. With him back in her life, I could be dispensed with—thank you very much! Perhaps unsurprisingly for someone involved in amateur dramatics, she had played her part very well—and so had I, albeit unwittingly. She had been playing a role in order to give me and her ex a certain impression—whereas I had been genuinely interested in her. And then the penny dropped! Her strong 'adaptive child' reading was a clue that I had missed—*that I had wanted to miss*! She even said that she loved pretending and that it was 'great'! But even at that stage, I was too involved to really hear her words and to tread with any sense of caution.

I'm convinced that I've been 'played' but I decide not to challenge her about it, as it would be her interpretation of events against mine. I assume she will now stop her hugs when we happen to be at the same dance. But on this, I'm proved wrong. For she still stops me whenever she sees me to give me a long, warm hug, right in the middle of the dance floor, quite irrespective of the other dancers around—and she continues to do so, whenever our paths cross. I really appreciate this as it suggests that she still likes me after all.

Unless, of course, she's simply maintaining the deception.

I'll never know.

But I choose to think the best of my great pretender.

9. Thinking out Loud
2004

"Jamie, how do you fancy teaching *The Philosophy of Religion*?" Hazel quips.

"Pull the other one!" I quip back. "It's not 1st April!"

But Hazel, my RS colleague, is serious. "Sometimes you're as daft as a brush! Half my GCSE group have asked me if they can do RS for 'A' level in the next academic year—that's fifteen of them!

"And they all want to do the philosophy and ethics course. I know that you'd want to do the philosophy paper and I'd prefer to do ethics myself. So Bob's your uncle!"

I'm amazed, though not actually that surprised. Hazel is an excellent teacher and became the No. 2 in the RS department, when Mr Milburn decreed that all pupils in Years 9 and 10 had to do a GCSE short course in RS. A few students from each year then opted to continue with the GCSE full course. Word soon got around about Mrs Kendall's teaching and the interesting topics on the course. Within a few years, she had a full classroom.

I'd had little to do with this GCSE success story, apart from being a supportive head of department. But now I'm going to be a beneficiary of Hazel's hard work and inspirational teaching as I take on my third 'A' level: sociology, psychology and now the philosophy of religion. I still have to teach the GCSE short course to four classes of Year 9 and 10 pupils, which includes some very disruptive characters. The blackboard jungle may have turned into a whiteboard jungle due to Mr Blair's reforms. But it's still a jungle—at least with some classes.

*

Now that my personal religious nightmare is well behind me, I relish the opportunity to revisit my old intellectual stamping grounds via the philosophy of religion. This time, I do not have the personal need to prove or disprove the existence of God. I now have a degree of objectivity that allows both myself and the students to come to our own conclusions—so long as their written answers demonstrate an adequate knowledge of various thinkers' arguments. Thinkers such as Socrates, Plato and Aristotle; Augustine, Aquinas and Kant; Kierkegaard, Hume and Nietzsche; Darwin, Freud and Sartre—among many others.

The syllabus also provides the opportunity to examine issues and arguments that evangelical Christians have never taken seriously (99); namely, Thomas Aquinas' classic 'proofs' of God, which include the cosmological, teleological and ontological arguments (100). When we come to the debate about *Theodicy*—the justification of God in the face of suffering and evil—I am back on familiar territory. But personally, I am no more persuaded to support the 'God thesis' now, than when I had firmly rejected it two decades previously.

The syllabus is broad-based and promotes the consideration of scientific, sociological and psychological approaches to religion. In science, we consider Darwin and evolution, Richard Dawkins' *The God Delusion* (101) as well as *String Theory* and *The Goldilocks Effect* (102) debated by leading physicists. In sociology, Marx's view of religion as *The Opium of the People* is an important critique. So is Norris & Inglehart's concept of *existential security*, which is the foundation of their world-wide survey that shows that religion prospers where populations have little such security, but that secularisation erodes religious belief where people feel relatively safe, such as in Western Europe [103]. In psychology, the anti-religious views of Freud and the pro-religious views of Carl Jung are discussed and debated within Year 13 classes. As evidence of 'wider reading', I introduce Attachment Theory's religiously neutral idea of 'God' providing a safe haven and a secure base for believers. For non-believers like myself, I see religion functioning as a substitute attachment—a necessary fantasy constructed to fulfil the psychological needs of tribes, nation states, individuals and other social groupings.

Most of the groups that Hazel and I teach contain a wide range of student views, including convinced atheists, uncertain agnostics, committed Christians and reflective Muslims. Despite our differences, we all share a willingness to discuss and debate with flexibility and respect. Most students also study either psychology or sociology, or both, so some learning is reinforced. In the philosophy of religion, discussions can be wide-ranging—so it's very much enjoyed by both the students and myself as we 'think out loud' together.

*

The results of the first group to go through the one-year AS course are a little disappointing, and none of them stay on for the full 'A' level course. As teachers, we realise that we need to go to more examiner's meetings before we quite understand what is required for exam success. Re-armed with this new information, the following year's group encounters no such problems and they all stay on for the two-year course, achieving results on or above their target grades in the process. It's gratifying that several go on to study philosophy at university.

As Hazel and I reflect on these achievements, we look back to the bad old days of RE's Cinderella status amid the blackboard jungle. I realise how fortunate I've been to join a school where there was a need for a new sociology teacher and then later, a need for psychology and philosophy & ethics in a growing sixth form. I can hardly believe the road I've travelled from those early dark days to now being the head of a department with nearly a hundred students taking either an AS or a full 'A' level course in the three subjects I'm responsible for.

Amid this intense level of reading, preparation, teaching and marking, I have still managed to learn to dance reasonably well and spend several evenings each week on the decadent dance floors of the east Midlands and beyond. It's taken some time to achieve but after my difficult years of post-religious trauma, I can wholeheartedly add modern jive dancing, psychology and 'A' level teaching to my list of passions, which already include Coventry City, Attachment Theory and chart therapy. But I *still* don't have a long-term girlfriend or partner—let alone the prospect of a marriage—which is what, in an ideal world, I would really like.

But it's not an ideal world, I tell myself, thinking out loud.

10. Emerging Passions: Review

i.   When I applied for and accepted the post as teacher of RE in my new, secular, state school, I half-realised I was heading for trouble (5.1). Not only that the pupils would be rougher and tougher compared with my previous independent school but that being responsible for RE throughout the school would be an albatross around my neck. And so it was. I hated it but I was stuck with it. That's what I was being paid to do. From an Attachment perspective, this suggests that I had 'merged' my identity so strongly with religion that it was nigh on impossible for me to assuage the pain triggered by the continual reminders [104]. At the school's pre-Christmas sing-song, I found the words of the carols impossible even to mouth, let alone sing—as nearby staff and pupils gave me disapproving looks.

ii.   It also makes sense that the anxious-ambivalently attached, such as myself, are more prone to 'merge' due to their tendency to shift from one extreme to another, dissolving personal boundaries in order to be 'one' with the object of their affection or devotion. I always felt that having to teach religion, after having decisively rejected it, felt like 'dragging a bad marriage around with me'; although I'd never been married! But I'd been more emotionally 'engaged' to religion than I had been to Sophie, and the process of leaving it was by far the most difficult task, with its long-lasting and most bitter after-taste.

iii.   In order to free myself from this albatross, I started to humanise and democratise RE through the questionnaire and poster approach—the less RE looked and felt like traditional religion, the better I could cope with it. In this respect, I was fortunate that RE had little or no status at the school when I arrived, for it meant that I had the freedom to change things in a way that helped both me and, I believe, the pupils.

iv.   Due mainly to the wisdom and generosity of Mr Milburn, the school acted as a 'haven' for me in those early years. Not the 'safe haven' of a secure attachment, because I didn't feel very safe being sworn at by pupils or by their threats to 'nut' me. My limited ability to control difficult classes added to my anxieties. Yet, it was a 'haven' from the sea of isolation and loneliness, had I remained at home without meaningful work to occupy me each day. Fighting for your life, whatever the situation, focusses the mind enormously. One's own existential angst tends to quickly recede when trying to cajole a disruptive Year 8 class into doing a modicum of work on a dismal Friday afternoon.

v.   My difficulty with classroom control in those early (and even later) days no doubt stemmed from my lack of a poorly developed critical parent figure, as Maggie had described (4.2). The fact that I had difficulty surface-acting such a figure only made matters worse (5.2 and below).

vi.   By the time I arrived at the blackboard jungle (5.1), I was suffering from intellectual as well as emotional trauma, following my intense reading during the latter stages of my religious life (3.7-9). Throughout the 'Francesca' and 'Coventry City F. A. Cup' years, I didn't read a single book. All I could manage were Coventry City match programmes and *The Sun* newspaper. I had no idea whether academic books were ever going to be important in my life, or whether they were the just the unwanted skeletons of my years in the religious wilderness.

vii.   Therefore, Mr Haigh's invitation to do some serious thinking in the form of 'A' level sociology (5.2) was both a revelation and a challenge—and inspired me out of my 'dogmatic slumbers'. He had read my CV and drawn his conclusions in a way that I couldn't, as I didn't want to look into my religious past at all. At my previous school, I had been keen to connect Christian moral theories, such as the sanctity of marriage, to some sociological data. But instead of biting off his hand with his offer, I was cautious in the extreme. The only rationale I can give for this is my lack of self-confidence, and my continuing intellectual trauma, that being merged with religion had bequeathed to me. I have Mr Milburn to thank in helping me overcome the former, and Mr Haigh for springing me out of the latter. They both believed in me far more than I believed in myself.

viii.   Teaching 'A' level sociology proved to be the start of my post-religious reconstruction of an alternative world-view to religion. Instead of seeing the world in terms of 'the saved' and 'the damned'—or in terms of the moral, the immoral and the amoral—I started to see the world in terms of social forces: economic (Marx), hierarchical (Durkheim) and popular (Weber). Sociology was starting to replace the systematic theology that had once held my world-view together. Now, without a so-called 'infallible Bible' creating anxiety, my only need was for well-conducted research, the establishment of facts and the need to sift an array of perspectives in order to arrive at justifiable conclusions. This is the process of social science methodology, in contrast to the mere affirmations of theological speculation.

ix.   The 10,000-word thesis that I produced was not a requirement of my MA course, or even a preparation for a further degree, despite my tutor's suggestion. It simply represented my need to develop a coherent view of the social world, using the research and theories of both sociology and psychology. My new psycho-social understanding of the world was starting to replace my religious world-view, and my new school was starting to take over the role of a secure (institutional) attachment that religion had hitherto provided.

x.   In my mind, mainstream macro-sociology took over from the broader religious themes of God, the world and the church—whereas psychology, TA and Goffman's Interactionism had much more useful things to say than St Paul about the inner workings of the human psyche and the way people interact with others. In particular, I found the following themes from micro-sociology [105] most illuminating about my life up to this point:

xi.   *Impression management*: As an evangelical Anglican minister, I felt that I was *always* duty-bound to create a positive impression, as that was a core element of one's witness to Christ. The clerical collar as a symbol of one's 'slavery to Christ' meant that one could not escape this obligation. I was, therefore, always aware of having to manage my impressions wherever I was and whatever I was doing. In my new school, I only had to impression-manage in certain situations—mainly in the classroom and with certain staff. The burden was therefore far less onerous. Away from work, I didn't feel the need to impress or manage myself at all!

xii.   *Front- and back-stage acting*: As an evangelical minister, I felt that my ministry always had to be front-stage and upfront. Only on rare occasions did I venture backstage, for example, with some innocent and spontaneous dancing at a church weekend where dancing was prohibited. Only once did I feel that backstage was a 'dark side'—in my temptation with Sophie (3.4) during teacher training, before we eventually got together. In Freudian terms, my superego (front-stage) was in overdrive, denying or repressing my back-stage potential (id). In TA terms, this suggests that I did indeed have a critical parent figure but that my criticisms were inward and self-directed in order to keep a lid on the mixed bag of my real self that remained in a repressed state [106].

xiii.   *Surface and deep acting*: As an Anglican, I disliked the wearing of clerical robes at services because I felt they represented an 'act' that I was putting on, that didn't correspond to my 'real' self. Apart from that, however, I had virtually no awareness of the distinction between the two. For the whole of my religious life, I was engaged in 'deep acting'. I didn't know where the boundaries of my 'real' self-ended—and those of religion began. I was hardly aware of a 'real' self as I was religious through and through—like 'Blackpool' through a stick of rock. But unlike the annoyed worker at the Blackpool rock sweet factory [107], I had never sworn a single time in my twenty religious years—despite being annoyed quite often. In my post-religious life, however, I knew that my classroom persona was a 'surface' act, which I could leave behind when out of school. I did not need to 'deep-act' any more—which was pure relief!

xiv.   *False self*: I can now see that for the whole of my religious period, I was living a false, inauthentic life—trying to be someone that I wasn't. The demanding nature of Christianity means that by 'giving your life to Christ', you really don't have a life of your own—the New Testament is quite clear about this. It's one of the few things that Jesus and St Paul agree about! For those who are securely attached in childhood through warm, loving parents, this may not be such a problem as they are psychologically rooted in a good, nurturing place [108]. But for the ambivalently attached who feel they need 'to give their all' to earn such security, the end-game is the loss of self. That is the main reason why my animosity remains towards any 'total commitment' to a God or religion. I almost lost my mind trying to justify a religious world-view that was, to me, intellectually untenable.

xv.   The establishment of TA in the classroom and then 'A' level psychology in the sixth-form (5.3-4) were two further strokes of luck for me, although brought about in part by their intrinsic interest and by my authenticity— with no 'deep acting' and little 'surface acting' needed. It was *exactly* what I wanted to be doing and teaching at that time.

xvi.   When my school life was developing so positively for me in the mid-90s, my social life continued to be difficult (5.5), first through the departure of Mike to the other side of the world and then through my inability to 'mingle' at social events. I was thoroughly inept at 'passing time' with people I didn't know and I needed social occasions to be purposeful if I were to remain interested.

xvii.   Through my discovery of *Ceroc* dancing (5.6), I found that sense of purpose: pop, dance and women all in one place. In a very real sense. I was rediscovering and developing another important aspect of my teenage life that I had sacrificed on the altar of Christianity at the age of sixteen. To a large extent, it became, and has remained, my main social outlet. I was gradually and painstakingly getting my pre-religious life back again—and then developing it.

xviii. As for my various relationships (5.5-8), the link between sex and love had already been broken for me by Karla four years earlier (3.9). This meant that I could enjoy sexual adventures without feeling emotionally overwhelmed. I had also become strong enough to end relationships, without only being on the receiving end of rejections. However, as I found out with Maisie and Amber (5.6-8), I could still be very vulnerable if I thought someone was offering me a relationship as well.

xix. With Georgie (5.7), I found myself in a completely new situation that I didn't understand. Had I done so, I might have treated her better, rather than keeping her 'hanging on' and in distress at my ambivalence. It was only much later that I realised that she saw me as her saviour, in much the same way that I had seen Francesca as *my* saviour, a decade previously. Of course, we were both needy, which made matters more complicated, and my inability to be a competent lover caused us both disappointment and, for my part, concern, after Maggie's analysis. For the period of our monthly dates, I tended to see her as an independent adult who could make up her own mind rather than the vulnerable person she was, being emotionally dependent on me to a degree that I never appreciated. Consequently, she hung on and ended up getting very hurt, which I very much regret.

xx. Teaching the philosophy of religion at 'A' level (5.9) gave me the chance to do some adult and relatively objective thinking about important issues that, in my religious life, I had undertaken in an immature, desperate and one-sided manner. Having already immersed myself in two social sciences ensured that I was now thinking and teaching from a broad intellectual base.

xxi. The philosophy of religion also had its counterpart in my teenage life; namely, my early reflections on the meaning of life with the songs of Bob Dylan and the *Selected Poems* of T.S. Eliot as my inspiration. I tend to think of my pre-religious teenage identity as: Coventry City, pop and girls; whereas 'reflective thinking' was, in fact, an important aspect, although the latest to develop, and was soon hijacked by my attachment need for evangelical religion. Now, along with *Ceroc* dancing, I was

231

coming to feel that the whole of my teenage potential was being realised, even if somewhat late in the day.

xxii.   It's clear with hindsight that both *Ceroc* and school were providing me with substitute (institutional) attachments as a secure base for my adult life. I didn't realise this at the time, as the only real attachment I was consciously looking for was a romantic female partner—preferably to marry! Nevertheless, although there were many attractive and interesting women at *Ceroc*, there did not appear to be one for me, despite a number of interesting adventures. Little did I know at the time where all this would lead: to romantic foreign travels perhaps? Yes! But only after a series of mid-life crises had shaken my world and had challenged me, once again.

*

To support positive mental health:

1. Support your own mental health, and that of others, by being aware of the damaging and stressful experiences that may have, in the past, contributed to various erratic or distressing behaviours. For example, the way you treat various partners, potential or real. The problem is that when suffering mentally yourself (however mildly), it's impossible to see inside another person's head to truly understand their point of view—because your own troubled mind is so self-focussed. At the same time, this is such a common impasse that there's no need to beat yourself up about it. But go easy with other people too! Try to be understanding, empathetic and non-judgemental, both towards yourself and others—so that good love doesn't turn bad.

2. Positive mental health can also be developed by being aware of and appreciating those people and circumstances in your life that are working well for you. It's all too easy to focus on the negative things in one's life, which results in the positive things being overlooked.

3. On a day-to-day basis, it can be helpful to look out for such issues as our impression-management, surface and deep acting and living out a false-self. It's virtually impossible NOT to manage our impressions—we do

so with virtually every person we meet in order to facilitate pleasant social relations. The problem is when we don't or can't distinguish these impressions from our authentic self. Therefore, someone who is continually posting only glamorous impressions of themselves on social media may come to believe that this represents their actual life—and a conflict may arise within, between the impressions and the more humdrum reality.

4. A similar situation may occur for all those people who work in the service sector and who, over time, confuse their smiley 'have-a-good-day' persona with their 'normal' self. They may end up deep-acting a false-self and lose their grip on their own identity. The same can be true for any individual who becomes deeply attached to any institution including work and religion.

5. The goal in social relations for positive mental health should be to be as authentic as you can be in any situation. This is not always possible but focus on those friendships that allow you to be comfortable being your real self. Hopefully, this will include a partner, if you have one.

Chapter 6 ~ Mid-Life Crises
1997–2001

1. A Curious Crisis

1997–9

It has just been announced from Paris that Diana, the Princess of Wales, has died.

It's difficult to take in.

I was already up in the early hours, unable to sleep. Made myself a cup of tea and a slice of toast, and turned on *Sky News* while marking a few essays. I soon put my pen down when it's announced that Diana has been injured in a car crash. I hope it isn't serious. But it is.

My godson, Ed, almost 15, is asleep upstairs. At 6 o'clock, I hear him stirring and take him a cup of tea—and the news. Ignoring the tea, he shoots downstairs, where we watch the unfolding drama together.

Like the assassination of President Kennedy in 1963, it's an event about which millions of people will always remember their actual location and experience at the time. From then on, it's wall-to-wall media coverage for the whole week and it's difficult to find a TV channel that's not about Diana. I have never met Diana in person but, like many others, I feel as though I have! Diana's charisma and her huge media exposure have seen to that. I had read Andrew Morton's book, *Diana: Her True Story* [109] and had identified her as being ambivalently attached due to her emotionally deprived childhood and her extreme mood swings both before and after her marriage to Charles. I could empathise with her. She reminded me of Francesca because of her height, her stunning good looks and those warm, penetrating eyes that fill your heart and soul with love. At dance, we are all shocked by the events in Paris and although most of us keep on dancing, both numbers and enthusiasm are down. A month later, I meet up with Georgie (5.7) and my hopes are raised once more for a long-term relationship, hopefully leading to permanence.

*

Mainly by myself, and occasionally with Georgie, I spend many evenings dancing modern jive to late '90s pop, such as the Mavericks' *Dance the Night Away*, Cher's *Believe* and Sash's *Mysterious Times*. In Grantham and Nottingham, there are dance groups where we all know each other and we travel the dance circuit together to dance *Ceroc*. The scene is slowly changing. More groups are springing up run by new franchises, and *Ceroc* itself becomes a franchise, with modern jive becoming the generic name for a dance that is a cross between rock 'n' roll and salsa. Together, we seek out new venues—here a Nottingham nightclub where we can dance modern jive, and there a Singles dance that we can, more or less, take over. We are mostly single ourselves— apart from the coupling-up, uncoupling and recoupling of course, such as Georgie and myself—from whom I eventually uncouple for good.

At most dances, I'm the last to leave the dance floor at 12.00 or 1.00, unless I'm in a relationship and we dance our way to an early bed instead. These are indeed mysterious times; for example, Sammy who sits on my knee for a snog at the nightclub while introducing me to her husband who also has a girl on his knee: "We have an open marriage, you see…" Then there's the tall, blonde Evie, who is the first girl to kiss me in the middle of a dance routine before asking me for a date—to which she fails to turn up! I was not amused and I didn't go near her again. However, there's also Katie and Angelique who are both sensible, reliable and caring and who become good friends and sources of good advice. As the millennium approaches, there's Suzie from Derby, with whom I have an on-off relationship for a few months, although it's nothing like as emotionally charged as my relationship with Georgie.

And then there's Ingrid…

*

I first set eyes on Ingrid at a Leicester nightclub that local modern jivers attend—so our Nottingham group decide to check it out. To me, Ingrid stands out in a curious sort of way—for she has a confident, almost business-like demeanour, her sharp navy outfit and rimless glasses contrasting with her striking, blonde, shoulder-length hair. I'm attracted but I assume that she would only be interested in well-built, confident guys, which I'm definitely not!

238

Nevertheless, we enjoy quite a few dances and I admire her Angelina Jolie lips close up, as we establish some sort of rapport.

It's over a month later when I bump into her again, as her Leicester group comes up to Nottingham for a Saturday night's dancing. Again, we seem to gravitate towards each other, but something is different. I'm curious and ask her if she wants to talk.

"Can we go for a walk?" came her request, almost at the point of tears. "But it will take you out from the dance."

"That's no problem—the music wasn't any good anyway…but something seems to be troubling you."

There's a very long, almost embarrassing pause, as though I've hit a raw nerve. I have. Eventually, she regains enough composure to speak.

"Jamie, you're the first person I'm telling this to but I had to tell *someone*. You see, my husband and I recently split up, and I told him a pack of fibs about why I wasn't happy."

"Go on…"

"This bit is really difficult… Okay, the *real* reason why I left was because I was in love with a person at work—a girl! I fell for a gorgeous young Asian woman, and she fell for me. But then her family found out and all hell was let loose—so she's left work and left me. So I'm in my own hell-hole right now."

There's a sharp intake of breath as gay relationships are well outside of my experience. But I do recall my own hell-hole in Desolation Row after Francesca had left—so I could empathise to an extent.

"Have you ever had such feelings for women before?"

"Sort of—when I was a teenager, my best friend and I had a 'thing' and we messed about a bit. But we soon got swept along into going with boys and forgot all about it. And I do like men…well, some of them. But I like women too. I think I must be bi-curious."

We carry on walking and talking for an hour or more, during which time she hooks her arm into mine. We part with a long hug, and she thanks me for listening to her without judging.

Later that week, Ingrid phones me to chat some more—but she also mentions that she needs a break. Would I be interested in going with her to a long dance-weekend on the Isle of Wight?

"I mean as friends, of course. But I'd be happy to share a chalet with you—with separate rooms."

"Yes, I'd love to—I could do with a break myself. And we do get on well…"

Of course, true to form, I'm somewhat overwhelmed by her suggestion—and wonder what might transpire in a seaside chalet by ourselves. And I start to notice afresh her fulsome lips and tight white blouses. In the event, we spend a long time chatting on the drive down about her sexuality—and mine. During the weekend, most other dancers seem to regard us as a 'normal couple' as we spend a lot of time together. And I do raise the possibility of us coupling up but she gently resists the suggestion. Other than that, we enjoy a great weekend and, upon our return, she's soon on the phone to thank me, yet again, for supporting her through her bi-curious identity crisis.

"Jamie, I know you like rock 'n' roll music, and I do too. So I'm wondering if you'd like to go to see *Buddy the Musical* at De Montfort Hall. It's meant to be good. It will be my treat—a sort of 'thank you' present."

I laughed: "I'd love to go. I've seen it several times before, so I know it's a great show. It's *Buddy brilliant*, in fact!"

*

Two weeks later, we meet at De Montfort Hall in Leicester, and Ingrid is looking the best I've seen her in a long while. I wonder if she's reconvened her relationship with the Asian lady—but she says not.

"I'm just about coming to terms with who I am—thanks to friends like you."

For the rock 'n' roll evening, she's ditched her business-like look and is wearing bright colours, including a blue and gold rock 'n' roll jive skirt—as I'd told her there'd be dancing in the aisles at the end of the show. She's in a very flirtatious mood and through most of the show, we sit close to each other, holding hands and with lots of smiley eye contact. How I'd love to kiss those Angelina Jolie lips! But there's no way I'm going to risk the friendship we have. For she had made herself clear on the Isle of Wight weekend, and I've come to accept that nothing is likely to change.

As the show builds towards its exuberant conclusion, she gets me up dancing in the aisle, before others join in—and I can't help noticing how high her skirt flares up as she whirls and twirls—but at least she's got matching underwear! As the aisle starts to get packed, we dance increasingly close to each other.

"Jamie, this is absolutely brilliant! I don't want it to stop! You'll come back for a coffee, won't you?"

Which, of course, I do.

We hold hands for much of the way back to her house, our fingers tightly interlocking. Upon our arrival and putting both arms around my neck, she kisses me full on, while wrapping a leg around mine. The kissing is prolonged and gets deeper, as my hands find their way to the flared skirt and the matching underwear.

With both of us half-undressed, she grabs my hand and leads me upstairs to her immaculately decorated pink and white bedroom, where the passion continues into the night and the early morning. In our post-coital cuddle, I start to reflect: "So then—what was *that* all about?"

"It's about me liking you very much—and I was curious what it would be like with you."

"Obviously, I know how you fancy the unavailable so I wanted to make the unavailable, available… But it's only a one-off—you do know that?"

"Yes, I do know that and that's okay. I'd always been aware that if we ever got together, it would be a one-off. But I always wanted to taste your lips and feel your body beautiful next to mine. And now I have!"

"So I guess we're *both* curious," came Ingrid's riposte, "but in different ways. *You're* curious about *unavailable* women, while *I'm* curious about *available* women! Ha ha!"

*

After that evening, we more or less go our separate ways. We always have a dance and a quick catch-up if we happen to be at the same dance venue. And if I see her dancing or talking with another young woman, I give her a knowing wink and she smiles back.

Little did I know it, but this was to be the last of my romantic adventures before the onset of my own major crisis of middle-life. But first, there's a party to be had!

2. It's Party Time!
December 1999

It's party time! It's music time! It's dance time!

For my 50th birthday, I push the boat out and have a big party! By now I have accumulated enough friends and acquaintances to fill a moderately-sized Nottingham ballroom. Almost 100 guests turn up, in three distinct groups: family and long-standing friends, dance friends and school colleagues. I want them to mingle, so I've been thinking how I might engineer this.

After a hot buffet has been consumed, I've arranged a beginner's dance lesson for (hopefully) everyone, and I specifically encourage my teacher-colleagues to get out of their cliques and off their seats and join in the fun—and most of them do. Ed has brought a live band from his sixth-form and they play their jazzed-up dance music for an hour, before a DJ takes over till midnight.

*

It is only my second birthday party since my 21st had been sabotaged by Celia breaking off our engagement a few days beforehand (3.2). I'm not really a party animal, preferring one-to-one conversations with friends, and I was happy to let my 30th pass by as it brought me up with a jolt—that I was about to enter middle-age! For my 40th, I had enjoyed an evening meal out with a dozen friends and colleagues. But now that I had discovered modern jive dancing, there was only one thing to do—book a ballroom for a big dance bash!

My parents are well into their eighties and do not attend. As for my brother Nigel, a dance party is so much his vision of hell that there's no chance of him turning up—but he wishes me well. I'm pleased that my godson Ed is here with his mother; Curly and his wife from way back when (1.3); as well as Maggie, my long-standing counsellor and friend, and her partner. Several of my Coventry City friends are here, together with twenty colleagues including Kevin Milburn and Hazel Kendall. Of my women dance friends, I'm happy to see Maisie and Ingrid along with Katie, Angelique and many others—most with boyfriends in tow. Paul, who had introduced me to *Ceroc* some three years previously, is also here with his video camera, but Georgie stays away.

*

The dancing, drinking and chatting continue till midnight. There's been a fair bit of mingling going on and it's pleasing for me that some of my friends have met others in the flesh rather than just by hearsay at our one-to-one conversations. I manage to have a word with most people individually, and also grab a dance or two with my various exes.

I receive many birthday cards with generous comments written inside. Presents are in abundance, many of them bottles, and some Coventry City related. But three are artistic: two framed prints from Jack Vettriano's collection: *Dance Me to the End of Love* from Angelique and *The Singing Butler* (Vettriano's signature painting) from Katie. Plus a book of his work from Ingrid [110]. I'm no art fan but I do like Vettriano's work. His attraction for me are his themes of dancing, decadence and popular culture—a reference to Vettriano's teenage roots (50s and 60s) that I wish had been mine! Paul's birthday gift is also appreciated when, at the end of the evening, he opens his video camera, takes out the cassette and hands it to me. I now have a valuable record of the evening, which I view over and over again in the days leading up to Christmas.

The week following the party, I receive many 'thank you' notes—the general theme being that it's the best party that many of my guests have ever attended. And coming from seasoned party-goers such as Curly and Joanna, that's one huge compliment. I can live on this for quite a while!

*

Except I don't...

It's now Christmas Eve and I'm still on a high from my 50th party.

But little do I know that this is to be the highest point of my dance revolution and that things will never be the same again.

Within twenty-four hours, I would realise that my dance party was definitely over.

3. Christmas Requiem

It's Christmas Day—and I'm off to my parents.

I'm taking all my 50th birthday cards to show them, as well as a selection of presents, including the Vettriano pictures. It will give us something to talk about, help fill the conversational and emotional vacuum that has existed between us for as long as I can remember.

*

Once off the motorway and into the leafy outer suburbs of Coventry, I admire the Christmas light displays that struggle to penetrate the cool morning mist. Still buzzing from my party, I have a good feeling about today. I'm feeling Christmassy and can almost smell the pale cream sherry that will be offered when I arrive.

As I pull up outside my parents' bungalow, I notice that there are no lights on, which is strange.

I start to make my way around the back but suddenly Mum opens the front door and beckons me in. That's strange too.

"Come in, Jamie, and go into the back room. Your dad's asleep and I want to talk to you."

Now *everything* is feeling strange, as there are no cards or decorations up. None at all.

"Jamie, I've some bad news to tell you. Very bad news… Your father is ill. Seriously ill. He's been diagnosed with something like Parkinson's disease."

"It's not Parkinson's, but it's similar—I can't remember the details."

"How serious is serious?" I enquire.

"He's been given a year to live at most, and it could be much less than that."

"Does he know? How long have you known?" Questions sear through my head.

"Yes, he knows and he's taken it stoically. Sometimes we're both a bit tearful. It was our diamond anniversary only two months ago—you were there for the meal."

"Does Nigel know?"

"Yes, he knows. We told him not to tell you because we wanted you to enjoy your party and not be worrying about us. The last time you had a party, it was spoilt by Celia breaking up with you (3.2). So we didn't want to spoil this one too."

Whatever the emotional disconnect between myself and Mum and Dad, they are genuinely caring people and I appreciated this thoughtful gesture. Mum is continually knitting garments for 'the schizophrenia society' and they've both worked for twenty years as volunteers in their local hospital.

But now I'm reeling, and this continues as we retire to the front room and I see Dad in his usual chair. He's looking pale and gaunt and unshaven. He never was a big man, but I can see his weight loss. His face is slightly contorted as if he has suffered a minor stroke—which he has. He opens his eyes.

"It's not a very happy Christmas, Jamie, but we only live once I suppose."

The whole day is spent in darkness, my dad wincing in occasional pain. There's not a hint that it's Christmas Day, and no cards or presents are given or exchanged. They don't want the TV on and they're not hungry. I get myself some beans on toast for lunch, which I eat alone in the dining room. It's unbearably bleak and sad. They don't even watch 'The Queen', which they've never missed before. It's all too much for me and I take myself off for a walk in the deepening afternoon gloom.

*

Alone on the walk, a strange feeling comes over me—*a slippage of time.* Two weeks previously (at my party), I was a happy, dancing Peter Pan. Suddenly, I feel like an old man with Father Time calling *me* in and the Grim Reaper sharpening his scythe *for me.* During my twenty-minute walk, thirty years pass by and I'm dying too. I'm keen to have a decent funeral, so I start to compose an Order of Service. I want songs by Roy Orbison and Bob Dylan and a reading from T. S. Eliot. As for Dad, something by Johann Strauss and an excerpt from a Beethoven symphony.

Before leaving for home, I give Dad a shave at his request and then have a cup of tea. I encourage both of them to eat a little, and promise I'll be back soon. It's a bad situation, and it being Christmas has made it much worse—by far the worst Christmas of my life. Back at home, I'm keen to put my thoughts on paper and I type out *two* Orders of Service for two funerals: Dad's and my own.

For although it's Dad who's dying, it's a Christmas Requiem for us both.

4. The Dancing Dies

My world has changed, within the space of a few hours on Christmas Day.

It feels like a seismic shift, the ground shaking under my feet and cracks opening up before me. The visible cracks are within the family structure, the shaking is within. None of us has experienced death at close quarters before. We've been lucky, but now our time has come.

*

I wonder if I should give up dancing out of respect for Dad—it hardly seems right. But my ceasing to dance will not help him, and self-imposed exclusion from my social life will not help me either—more likely, it will trigger my loneliness and depression. So I continue dancing through January and February, while Dad continues to decline.

However, I find that the more I dance, the less I enjoy it. It seems so superficial, with arms waving madly in the air, and to what purpose? For me it's lost its meaning. It doesn't touch me like it used to. It doesn't touch my soul or my sadness. I discuss this with Angelique, with whom I enjoyed a brief flirtation the previous year before we decided that we were best as friends. Angelique is a doctor in general practice, almost twenty years my junior—but she has a wise head on her young shoulders as well as a sympathetic ear. She suggests an alternative to dancing.

"Why don't we go to *Mahler's 2nd Symphony* in Lincoln Cathedral? It won't cheer you up, but it might connect with you better than dancing to pop."

She's right, it does. I'd never heard Mahler before—but I'm moved throughout by its themes, and in particular by the choral finale. *The Resurrection* symphony is not a requiem, but it feels as though it is. The next day I buy a CD to appreciate it again. I then start to buy other Mahler symphonies, which really suit my mood A week later, we go to Durham for the day. Angelique has never been before and with the bare trees and bleak cathedral, it seems the right place to be.

In March, we go to hear *Mozart's Requiem in D Minor*, a beautiful and profound work that I am familiar with. After this, I listen only to music for solemn occasions. In addition to Mahler and Mozart, there are Requiems by Faure, Cherubini, Berlioz and Verdi, which all inspire me, but Berlioz is the most profound and majestic. However, amidst the sadness of the Requiems, I occasionally attend a dance, thinking it may cheer me up. But I realise that I don't want cheering.

My father is now in terminal decline and has been moved to a hospice near their home. On one occasion when my brother Nigel visits, staff tell him of a potentially fatal accident that Mum almost caused when she pulled out from the drive without looking. So Nigel and I agree that Mum, at 84 and clearly disorientated, is not fit to drive anymore. Nigel removes the car keys from the bungalow and informs Mum. She's distraught at losing the car and with it, her independence—almost as much as losing Dad. In the end, she sees common sense, albeit reluctantly. From now on, it's the world of taxis for her. Her next-door neighbours are saints in terms of the help they provide for her when Nigel and myself can't be there.

In mid-May, I visit my father who is now very weak. He's in a private room and sitting up in his chair. We talk briefly about this and that, but I'm unable to tell him the things I'd like to—how grateful I'd been for the times when he would stick up for me when Mum was too demanding and his other kindly deeds. We would have both been embarrassed as we just didn't talk like that in our family. Before I leave, he asks me to put him back in bed. I pick him up, and he hardly weighs a thing. As I put him down, I kiss his forehead. I realise that I may never see him again. I don't.

*

The following Saturday, it's the F. A. Cup Final at Wembley in the afternoon, then in the evening, Angelique and I are going to hear *Verdi's Requiem* in Lincoln Cathedral—a strange sort of day. Upon my return home, there's a message on my answer-phone to call the hospice: my father had passed away in the middle of the evening, while I had been at the Requiem. By sheer coincidence, the very same day, Bernard Hitchiner, a family friend and Coventry

248

City administrator (who had obtained my Cup Final ticket), also died. My father is dead, a family friend is dead and football doesn't seem to matter anymore. With a funeral to prepare for and a mother who needs my support, it's also the day that the dancing dies.

5. The Last Goodbye

"You can't say that! You'll have us all in tears!"

*

As I park outside my parents' bungalow, I see that Nigel's car is already there. Mum is going about her usual chores, a bit wobbly on her feet, but keeping calm and carrying on. The three of us sit down together over coffee.

"Nigel, will you contact the funeral people, and then make a start on your dad's finances? I suspect they're in a mess."

"Jamie, I want you to help me with the service, as you've done this sort of thing before. A few years ago, your dad went to a funeral that was a bit different. It had no hymns, no Bible readings or prayers, but had a mix of classical and pop music, and an address about the man who had died. No sermonising. Your dad liked it, and said he would want a service like that."

"You mean a Humanist service?"

"Yes, that's it. Humanist. Can you arrange that?"

I pop into the hallway to get the Yellow Pages directory, to search under H.

"Here it is: *Humanist Association for Coventry & Warwickshire*. I'll give them a call."

*

Between the three of us, we agree that Dad would have four pieces of his favourite music: *Nimrod* by Elgar, *The Blue Danube* by Johann Strauss, Beethoven's *Pastoral Symphony 5th movement* and Handel's *Largo*.

We then talk about the tribute and Mum asks me to draw up a rough draft. It's not an easy task as Dad was a very retiring man and you never really knew what was going on inside his head. Definitely not an action man, despite his war years in the RAF. He always said he'd had 'an easy war' and only saw one dead German during his search and rescue missions over the North Sea. Although not close, I'm fond of Dad and write a tribute that expresses that, which I then give to Mum to read.

"You can't say that! You'll have us all in tears!"

I smile and suggest that that is rather the point of a funeral service—to express one's feelings about the deceased.

"Well, I don't agree so please change it and remove that emotional stuff!"

I show the same draft to Nigel and can anticipate his reaction: it is the same as Mum's. I'm outvoted 2:1 and rewrite the tribute in a more matter-of-fact, prosaic and stoical style. It's as dry as dust, but now approved by the censors! We each write our own card to put with the flowers.

Mine says: "Thank you for your kindness, the football and so much else. To a good dad and a lovely man. Much love, Jamie x."

Nigel's says: "Thanks Dad."

Mum's says: "What do you have to go and leave me for?"

Whilst understanding Mum's distress, I suggest that it sounds a bit harsh. She agrees and softens the tone. Mum asks if I will read out the tribute at the service. I want to do it, but I fear I'll break down in the middle. So we ask the official from the Humanist Association do the honours and to lead the rest of the service.

The funeral takes place at *The Heart of England Crematorium* near Nuneaton. The view of the green Warwickshire countryside from the large clear window behind the altar is especially fitting, as both Mum and Dad enjoyed many countryside trips together, complete with a 'tommy cooker' for a fresh cup of tea. The service goes well and it's a good turnout. I didn't realise how many friends and admirers Dad had.

Mum is sad but stoical. Nigel expresses no emotion. I'm heading for a breakdown.

6. Breakdown

Time continues to collapse. I'm 50 but I feel 80.
The clock ticks faster. Time is running out.

As the dust settles after my father's funeral, Nigel and I agree to visit Mum every Saturday, alternating with each other. She has wonderful next-door neighbours, but she will also have a visit from Nigel or myself every weekend. It's not something that either of us will particularly look forward to—due to our emotional disconnectedness—but it's our duty for at least a year, perhaps longer.

I'm not in the mood for dancing when I'm so unbearably sad and consequently, I'm starting to feel socially isolated once again. I console myself by listening to solemn Requiem music as that's the only music I want to hear. I'm sad about Dad, and Mum, and I'm also sad about myself—that I may have so little time left before my own funeral. Time is moving on and will soon run out, but I'm standing still…

In an attempt to relieve my mounting distress, I decide to get back on the dating scene. I agree to meet Amelia at a local pub—perhaps she will become the love of my life and save me from myself and my lonely existence! She sounded nice on the phone and her photo looks great! But when we meet face to face, my heart sinks. She's dismal and dowdy and nothing like the voice on the phone or the photo she had sent. I think she should be charged under the Trade Descriptions Act! I mumble a few things about my father having died and that I shouldn't be doing this. Then, without a second thought, I leave her standing in the pub. I'm right—I *seriously* shouldn't be doing this!

The following evening, Ed comes over to watch *Monday Night Football* on *Sky* and we chat about his 'A' levels and football. Next morning, I give him a lift to his school before setting off for mine. But after I've dropped him off, I'm gripped by a terrible thought: I'm due to be teaching *The Mid-life Crisis* to my Year 13 psychology group in an hour's time—but I can't do it! I'll break down! I'll be having a mid-life crisis in the middle of teaching about a mid-life crisis! In the past, various students have said that I'm a good psychology teacher because I've experienced so much myself—but there's no way I'm going to humiliate myself in front of the class! So I make a decision: I will drive home, phone the school and explain my absence. As always, Mr Milburn is very understanding: "Take off what time you need, Jamie. Send in what lessons you can manage, and we'll cover the rest."

I'm relieved and extremely grateful, and I book a doctor's appointment.

*

I manage to get in the following morning. It's a lady doctor. "How can I help?"

Once I start speaking, I pour it all out nonstop for fifteen minutes. She listens patiently to it all—my father's death, the requiems, the collapsing of time, giving up dancing, time running out, social isolation, my dating failures—then having to teach about a mid-life crisis! It all comes out in a breathless jumble—like being sick—a verbal and emotional mess.

She waits until I've finished.

"James, it seems to me that you're suffering from anxiety and depression. I will prescribe you a course of anti-depressants, and you should take three to four weeks off school. Come back to see me if you need to."

A huge weight is lifted off my shoulders—being able to open up and 'let it all out', to have a label attached to my condition and to be given medical permission to take time off school. I return home, already feeling lighter. I feel physically fit, I'm mentally alert—it's just my emotions I need to sort out and that won't happen overnight. I'm aware that being anxiously-ambivalently attached, I'm vulnerable in crisis situations to intense roller-coaster emotions. I accept that this is who I am—so I'm not too hard on myself. It comes with the territory—with my particular ambivalent-attachment territory.

I prepare what lessons I can and send them off to school with apologies to my students. Feeling freer and more relaxed, I decide to bring my scrapbooks up to date, especially about Dad's funeral. Then more chart-work that I've recently neglected. It's creative, fulfilling and therapeutic.

It gives me a better sense of who I am and where I have come from, psychologically speaking. So I now feel in a better place to think about what I might do and where I might go—before it's my turn to die. I then hit on a new idea—two, in fact. I shall visit Grantham town centre: first the bookshop and then the travel agents.

I'm starting to feel a revolution coming on!

7. Cultural Revolution
Autumn term, 2000

"We're going to Barcelona for Easter.
Where are you off to, Sally?"
"It's Egypt for Chuck and me—a Nile cruise."
"Nice one! We did Egypt last year—it was wonderful!"

A chance conversation overheard in the staffroom triggers a thought and lights
a fuse—it's a slow burning fuse, but it ignites my own cultural revolution!

*

I emerge from the bookshop with half-a-dozen *Icon* books [111]: Cultural Studies, Media Studies, Levi-Strauss, Muhammad, Chomsky and Wagner—all aspects of culture that I don't know a thing about. My culture and education hitherto has been white, British, Christian and rational. Convergent thinking. I'm suddenly restless to diverge! There's a big world out there!

My overheard staffroom conversation reminds me that I'd not been out of UK since my pilgrimage to L'Abri in Switzerland (2.5) in 1971—almost thirty years! I'm envious of the young staff who seem to go off anywhere and everywhere at the drop of a hat. Therefore, at the travel agents, I collect a pile of brochures and start to dream of adventures to far-off places.

*

Back home, I settle down with my books and brochures, I feel lighter in spirit mentally, though still depressed emotionally. It's a curious mixture. The 'collapsing of time' brought about by my father's death has raised a vital question—*how can I best fill the years I have left?* I have no doubt about the answer: explore the world, both intellectually and geographically! I have a new mission and at last there's a light at the end of my mid-life tunnel. However, there's a couple of immediate problems: having spent a thousand pounds on my party, I'm short on finances. And I've no one to travel with. So I have a hidden agenda; I'm still looking for a partner or can I travel the world alone? Okay, so my agenda is not so hidden! I temporarily resolve these problems by joining a singles' group that specialises in holidays and short breaks.

Feeling recovered enough to return to school, I now have plans to visit Paris in the summer with this group for a long weekend. We go via Eurotunnel and see the sights. I'm impressed by Notre Dame, I'm fascinated by the Montmartre district with its artists, the Moulin Rouge and its strip clubs and sex shops—plenty of decadence here! But the Palace of Versailles makes the greatest impact on me as I stroll in the gardens among the thousands of other tourists. For the first time since I was a teenager, I feel normal! A normal person doing what other normal people do on holiday. Up till this point in my life, my energy had been spent on religion—either being imprisoned by it or escaping from it, its influence having lingered on for many years after I had formally rejected it. But in Versailles, I'm pleased to be a part of mass tourism, for I feel that I've re-joined the human race! It's been a long time coming.

On the coach journey back to the UK, I get talking to Yasmin, a modern Iranian lady whose parents had fled the 1979 revolution. She's very interesting to talk to and I sense some *frisson*. So we meet up again in Nottingham where our relationship quickly becomes sexual—so much so, in fact, that our cultural conversations soon dry up. By the end of the summer, however, our fling has burned itself out as we are not in love. In any case, Yasmin has been taking a risk with me in case her parents found out. I think that I represented her rebellion against her parents' frequent attempts to arrange a traditional marriage for her. We agree to end things, with no hard feelings and with some happy memories. After another brief affair, I'm feeling even more like my normal self!

*

By now, I've definitely got the travel bug, but where shall I go next and with whom? As Islam is an important topic on the new GCSE RE course at school, I would like to experience an Islamic culture—within western Europe, if possible. Andalusia in southern Spain seems ideal, with its Moorish past. Angelique recommends a couple of holiday companies, such as *Explore Worldwide* or

Travelbag Adventures, that specialise in small group tours. She's been with these groups several times and speaks highly of them. As it happens, *Travelbag* are running a holiday to Andalusia during my October half-term. I'm nervous about meeting new people but nevertheless, I sign up and pay my deposit.

However, it's not unknown for revolutions to take unexpected turns, and my 'cultural revolution' is no exception.

8. Taking Off

Put On Your White Sombrero: Abba [112]

As the plane enters the clouds, I switch on my Walkman, relax and enjoy the uplifting harmonies of Abba, in this Spanish-sounding, feel-good song. Maybe I will meet a sweet senorita on this holiday to Granada! But as the majority of our party are from Hull and Grimsby, I'm not holding my breath [113].

*

I've been feeling more confident with my 'cultural revolution' taking off—so I return to the Monday night dance class in Grantham. As I pay my admission, I notice a dance-holiday brochure on the table for Granada in southern Spain. The October dates coincide with my half-term so I immediately cancel my *Travelbag* trip and book myself for a dance holiday with *Ceroc*!

After driving through the early hours, I'm as excited as a little child as I arrive at Stansted Airport just as dawn is breaking. It's almost 30 years since I'd flown and the airport atmosphere is fascinating, not least the new technology and the driverless trains that transport us to our plane. I'm intrigued by the relaxed demeanour of my fellow passengers at the terminal, considering we're all about to be cooped up in a flying sardine tin that could be terminal for us all if things go wrong. I'm a bag of nerves as we take off, relaxing only as the plane levels out and I tune into the uplifting sounds of Abba.

It's pleasantly warm as we arrive and settle in at our hotel, then set off for a tapas meal at a local restaurant. It's a wonderful treat of meats and other delicacies as the tapas trays keep on arriving. Sweet Malaga wine also keeps on arriving in my glass, so I enjoy a very merry time with my fellow dancers. For the following six nights, we hit the salsa bars of Granada, where there's a friendly atmosphere, with the locals and ourselves swapping various dance moves. After a couple of morning *Ceroc* classes, I drop out to discover the delights of Granada—particularly its leafy plazas and the Moorish *Albaicin* district with its whitewashed dwellings, labyrinthine streets and slender green cypress trees. Then on to the nearby *Plaza San Nicolas*, which provides breath-taking views over the *Alhambra Palace* and *Generalife Gardens*—the jewels in Granada's crown. I'm not a huge fan of palaces or gardens, but the open-air *Alhambra* is stunningly beautiful with its detailed Islamic patterns, geometric architecture, pools and courtyards. The *Generalife Gardens* are sumptuous and sparkling with their fountains, flowers and air of tranquillity. I'm delighted to visit them both again with the dance group later in the week.

*

Back on the dance-floor, there's a single lady, Sandy, who seems a bit taken with me, but I'm not taken with her. Anna's dancing interests me however—it's close-up, flirty and sexy—then she points out that her husband is only a few feet away! But she dances even closer so I assume they must have a reciprocal arrangement. It's true: modern jive can be 'sex on legs' at times!

On our final day, we all go for a lunch-time meal together—a set meal this time. After we've finished eating, I wonder what happens next. Twenty minutes later, I realise that nothing happens next, but everyone else keeps chatting away quite happily—except me. So I take my leave into the blistering afternoon heat. I make my way back to the *Albaicin* district where I see a young lady, the only person in an open-air cafe that overlooks the city's heat-haze. I ask if I may join her and we chat for over an hour before we wander back towards the *Alhambra*. Lotte is Dutch and a social science teacher like me, so we have plenty to talk about. She's attractive, with a sweet smile, a long blonde ponytail and without a boyfriend. Reluctantly, I realise there's too much of a generation gap—so after a farewell hug, we go our separate ways. She's the nearest to a sweet senorita that I meet.

Having returned to Stansted I'm homeward bound up the A1—and I'm almost expecting the nose of my car to lift off the tarmac, as I sing along with Abba once more. I'm happy to have rediscovered my flying wings and my dancing feet on this magical, atmospheric adventure.

My mid-life crisis appears to be over—my life is taking off once more!

9. Castles in the Sky

*She takes hold of my hand and places it on the top of her perfect apple-bottom
or 'the base of my spine', as she calls it.
"Now, whenever you do a 'drop', that's how I want you to do it!"*

Returning from Granada on a high, I'm full of energy and expectation when I step out onto the familiar dance floors of Grantham and Nottingham. It's been six months since Dad's funeral. I miss him, especially when I visit Mum every other week. But I'm not lost in sadness any more, and I'm off the anti-depressants. As the autumn nights close in, the dance scene is livelier than ever, with some new faces as well as familiar ones welcoming me back. My favourite dance partners seem flirtier than usual, so I'm confident that before long, I'll meet Miss Right or, being more realistic, Miss Almost Right. It's been a long time since my last proper relationship.

Of the newly arrived dancers, Casey immediately catches my eye at the Friday night freestyles. She moves and dances very easily and her stylish hair seems a cut above the rest—layered and shoulder-length at the back, and to one side at the front. I also notice there's no wedding ring on her ring finger and I later discover she's a GP at a health centre in Melton Mowbray—and a very single GP at that. I wait for my moment to ask her for a dance and right from the start, there's a connection. She's both vivacious and curvaceous and I can't help admiring her considerable cleavage on display. But it's her eyes that contain the chemistry for me.

She always wears black, usually long dresses, but occasionally a long split skirt—split to the top of her thigh and sometimes with a bare-midriff. Despite these distractions, it's still her eyes that entrance me. Whatever move we are doing, whichever way her body is facing, her eyes are always on mine. Sometimes, she needs a quick flick of the head to re-engage—but it's only a split second before our eyes are locked again. The first time we meet, we dance half a dozen dances straight off, which is not *Ceroc* etiquette. We do dance with others but we're soon back together and I realise there's a couple of moves she doesn't do with anyone else. They seem reserved for me. The first is where she allows her hand to linger around my neck before she brushes it very slowly across my cheek. It feels the most intimate of moves! Then there's the drops. She doesn't seem to do them with anyone else, but she tells me that she has a 'dodgy knee' (to which she gives a fancy medical name) and that she wants me to place my hand on 'the base of my spine' to support her properly. We practise it and she comes up with a huge grin on her face—I'm not at all convinced by her 'dodgy knee'! But I'm happy to do as many of these drops as she wants!

We also talk a lot—especially about her work as a GP, and about foreign travel, as I've just gained a taste for it, and she's a long list of locations she wants to visit, preferably not alone. Perhaps she's looking for a travel companion? I decide not to tell her about my religious past, in case she thinks I'm a bit weird. But I'm already imagining touring far and wide with Casey, and I start to make a mental list of common destinations that we'd both like to visit. I'm feeling my luck is about to change as she dances and talks with me so much. We even experiment with 'blind dancing' as our bodies feel so in tune with each other; we shut our eyes, dance closely and still get the moves right! We've also embraced a song that's often played at the dances we attend: *Castles in the Sky*, which was released earlier that year [114].

With Christmas over, I decide to ask Casey about going out together—or at least a joint travel adventure. At the New Year's Eve dance, we've just finished dancing to *Castles in the Sky* when she takes me to one side and sitting at a table, alludes to the song: "Jamie, do you ever question your life? Do you ever wonder why we're here?"

At last, I think to myself, *someone who's on the same wavelength as me! Surely, she must be interested!*

"Yes! All the time!" I eagerly reply. "I'm always thinking and analysing stuff! What about you?"

"In medical matters, yes, research is important. But as for the meaning of life, *analysis is paralysis!* Just thinking about things will get you nowhere. It's best just to believe and stay positive."

"Believe in what? I believe in Attachment theory: it's helped me understand my chaotic life!"

As a GP, I expect she'll know the rudiments of Attachment theory but she doesn't take it up.

Instead, she announces: "Believe in the Lord Jesus Christ and you will be saved [115]. I've started going to church recently with a Christian doctor from the health centre—and I've become a born-again Christian. But what about you? Are you saved? Did you know that Jesus can save you?"

~

I'm stunned into silence—I can't believe it! I want to cry!
"Oh tell me why do I keep building castles in the sky?"

10. Mid-Life Crises: Review

i.   I see the four years of 1996-9 as my *Peter Pan* years when I was living out, as an adult, the realisation of my teenage dreams: I watched Coventry City playing good First Division football to large crowds and *Ceroc* dancing was fuelling my interest in pop and providing me with a good social life, attractive women, relationships and sex (6.1-2). My reflective side was almost over-stimulated with my introduction of 'A' level psychology to the sixth-form. These were passionate years! In many ways, they reminded me of my teenage years of 1963-6 (1.7-2.2): football, pop, girls and T. S. Eliot—and with two historic media events to mark the changing times: the assassination of President Kennedy in 1963 and the death of Princess Diana in 1997. After almost two decades in the church, then a further decade in recovery (2-4), I now have some years in which to enjoy what I had previously missed out on when struggling in the long and dark night of my religious wilderness.

ii.   There were, however, a few negatives for me in the late 90s, although mostly unconscious:
1. Life was jam-packed and helter-skelter with little room for quiet reflection.
2. I was still searching for a life-partner, without success.
3. Like most (but not all) teenagers, I had no awareness of death. I was immortal.

iii.   Therefore, when I arrived at my parents' house on Christmas Day, to be informed about my father's terminal illness (6.3), I felt I was a runaway train hitting the buffers. By the time I drove home that night, I was experiencing two classic features of a mid-life crisis:
1. the sudden, brutal awareness of my own mortality
2. the overwhelming perception of time 'running out'

iv. The reaction of my brother Nigel and myself to the news about my father may appear inconsistent, given the emotional disconnect between ourselves and our parents that also exists between the two of us. However, in attachment terms, although my brother and I both had an insecure attachment with Mum and Dad, we still had an attachment of sorts—the physical aspect of which was about to be ended through our father's death. This meant for me that, for the time being, other substitute attachments had to take a back seat (6.4), primarily Coventry City and dancing [116]. Even though our attachment to Dad had never been strong, we were both sad that it was about to end. We both maintained our weekly commitment to Mum for two complete years after Dad's funeral. We both found Mum much harder to be with than Dad so our commitment was more from a sense of duty than from any emotional connection.

I had to smile when I read the three cards to be placed with Dad's flowers at the funeral (6.5): mine was in a 'caring parent' style (as per Maggie's Ego-gram of me); Nigel's two words were stereotypically avoidant and 'adult'; and Mum's was in 'critical parent' mode. I could have almost predicted them and they clearly symbolised the wide differences between us. None of us were ever 'close'.

v. My breakdown, when it came, contained two further elements that are common in reports of mid-life crises (6.6):
1. The creation of personal space for reflections of a new and challenging nature—in my case, time away from work.
2 The making of positive decisions about aspects of one's future—in my case, opening my life to a 'cultural revolution', which included a determination to travel abroad—if necessary, without a partner.

It is a feature of most reported mid-life crises that they contain both negative and positive elements, with new directions emerging from the relics of the past. In my case, the relic was my assumption that both myself and my parents would go on forever.

vi. As for mid-life crises in general, social scientists are very much divided. Carl Jung believed that such a crisis (like his own) was an essential stepping-stone to the process of *individuation* [117] that helps make people 'whole'. The Stage theories of Erikson and Levinson assume that some sort of crisis is necessary at each new stage of the life-course for people to progress from immature ways of being and move on to new growth. It was Daniel Levinson who popularised the idea of a mid-life crisis based on his sample of men where 80% had experienced some personal turbulence at about the age of 40 [118]. It is well known that sociologist Max Weber had a lengthy mid-life breakdown of over six years, from which he emerged as an intellectual giant [119]. In the contemporary world, sociologist Anthony Giddens claims that: *The phenomenon of the 'mid-life crisis' is very real for many mature adults today* [120]. However, he is careful not to specify what percentage of the population this crisis may afflict—and there is a good reason for this...

vii. The reason for Giddens' hesitance is probably due to the fact that the majority of contemporary psychologists see no sound research basis for a 'mid-life crisis' existing at all—except perhaps for a tiny minority of people. In most psychology textbooks, including dictionaries, there is no indexed reference to the term and Levinson's 80% result has not been replicated in other research. The lifespan psychologist, Helen Bee, in reviewing the evidence, suggests that white, middle-class men in professional occupations may be a sub-group that are more at risk of such a crisis [121], for which there may be a variety of reasons. Others suggest that the culture of youth in western Europe has helped popularise the concept due to our need to continually re-invent a more youthful version of ourselves in spite of—or perhaps because of—the aging process.

viii. The main reason for this virtual dismissal of the mid-life crisis is that the term has no precise definition: when is 'personal turbulence' or a 'transition period' or a 'stressful event' a mid-life crisis? Or can it be identified with a change or loss of employment, or a loss of or change of spouse, or a loss of family member through disagreement, divorce or death? It seems that the concept is too vague to be researchable. Therefore, people tend to label all sorts of adult setbacks as 'a mid-life

265

crisis'. Nevertheless, as Giddens correctly states, a *serious* crisis of great personal significance does affect many people in their mid-life.

ix. Attachment theory and literature are little different in this respect from more general psychology. There is no reference to the term in major Attachment textbooks. However, there is considerable discussion of the effect of stressful events on those securely, avoidantly and ambivalently attached. The overwhelming (and unsurprising) conclusion is that the securely attached cope much better with stressful life-events in adulthood than do the insecurely attached [122]. Furthermore, it is widely acknowledged in psychological literature that those who have a history of life-crises are vulnerable to experiencing more. I would certainly fit into this picture. After 'discovering' Attachment theory, I thought that life might be smoother for me thereafter. But I was soon forewarned that 'anxious-ambivalents' are especially vulnerable to emotional turbulence and that emotional crises, mid-life or otherwise, are in fact par for the course.

x. As a result of my breakdown and time off school, I was able to reflect about how I wanted to fill the 30 years that, hopefully, were left for me. My personal ambitions quickly emerged: wider cultural thinking and world-wide travel. But how to do it? That was the problem. With all my insecurities, there was no way I would suddenly transform into a globe-trotting, mountain-climbing, independent explorer.

I realised it would be a question of baby steps. Hence, my first trip was to Paris by train with a similarly aged group (6.7)—hardly Mao's Long March! My second trip, to Granada, was slightly more adventurous, with my first flight in 29 years to negotiate and an Islamic sub-culture of western Europe to experience (6.8). It certainly gave me a taste for more.

xi. Upon my return home, however, I quickly slipped into old ways with my dancing dalliance with Casey (6.9). I actually knew why I built *Castles in the Sky* because of the well-established propensity of anxious-ambivalents for fantastical thinking (4.6) in their attempt to make people and situations appear more promising than they actually were. But I still did it—I couldn't help myself, especially when in the company of such a sensuous lady—with mature and sensible 'Adult' thinking quickly going out the window—as the fantastical flight of Free Child imaginings took over!

xii. When my *Castles* came crashing down as Casey tried to 'save' me, I realised that although my mid-life crisis was past, I had a continuing crisis to address: my need to find a long-term partner with whom I could eventually live and establish a home together. This search led me into further cultural exploration and to more adventurous travel plans. Not Mao's Long March…more like Lenin's journey to St Petersburg—before my personal revolution was to eventually establish a new order.

*

To support positive mental health:

1. Almost by definition, it's difficult to navigate oneself in a crisis because many familiar landmarks have disappeared. Therefore, it's natural to keep repeating behaviours that you think will help—even if they don't. For me, it was both dating and dancing. For others, it might be continuance in social media or maintaining damaging friendships or behaviours such as alcohol or drugs—or something else. In such circumstances, it is important to be honest with oneself about what is working and what is not—and to cut out the latter.

2. In times of crisis, we need to nurture ourselves in small ways, like playing some favourite music, buying some favourite food—but not to build 'castles in the sky', imagining that some external source / Prince Charming / fairy godmother will come to rescue us. In the process of nurturing and rescuing ourselves, we can (and will) learn some important lessons as all personal crises will have happened for some reason or other, or more likely for several reasons.

3. As for mid-life crises in general, to have a wise confidante, therapist or GP to talk things through with (and/or prescribe anti-depressants if needed) is always helpful. A spouse or partner could play this role—except that one's relationship with someone so close may form part of

the crisis itself. Both partners may be too close to the proverbial trees to be able to see the woods or rainforest of a mid-life crisis.

Chapter 7 ~ Russian Revolution
2001–11

1. To Russia with Love
January 2001

"Attractive Russian ladies with traditional values seek mature British gentlemen for romance and marriage."
Apply: Eurocontact magazine.

I don't do New Year's resolutions but this year is different, in that I'm resolved to travel *and* hopefully meet a partner for life, or even a wife! I have come to the conclusion that dancing probably attracts more than its fair share of middle-aged singletons who have been damaged through inadequate parenting, like myself, or other negative life experiences—and *that* perhaps is the reason why, through dance, I've had several liaisons and various girlfriends, but nothing approaching a life-long partnership, or marriage. So I need to look elsewhere and the dating section of *The Guardian* is where I start. Initially, I scan the lonely hearts ads, but I want something different! So I look across to the dating agencies column, where I see the advert for *'Attractive Russian ladies'*.

I assume that by 'traditional values', it means that they aren't keen on divorce or on bed-hopping, which sounds good, as I want someone who will stay. I'm not sure whether 'mature' means 'committed', 'middle-aged' or 'with money', but in any case, I think I'll be okay on that one. 'Romance' I like and 'marriage' certainly suggests a life-long relationship. However, in the back of my head, I recall Maggie's opinion that, for me, a woman's availability might reduce my sexual interest (5.7). But hey ho—that was a complicated, multi-factored situation with Georgie, which I cannot allow to dictate my future. Anyway, it was only a 'suggestion' from Maggie—marriage to an attractive Russian lady might be just what I need!

*

I send off my £7.00 and the *Eurocontact* magazine arrives a week later. It's an exciting read, with hundreds of attractive-sounding ladies from all over eastern Europe wanting to meet men like—me! Most ads come with box numbers, addresses or telephone numbers—but just one comes with an email address. Having just obtained my first PC, I send off my first long-distance email. I'm astonished by the result as later that day, I receive a reply from Elena in St Petersburg, telling me quite a bit about herself—and a number of revealing photos of herself in a bikini at a Black Sea resort. I'm impressed and reply with (not so revealing) photos of myself. After corresponding with her daily for over a week, she tells me that her mum is very ill and needs expensive medicines that they cannot afford. Could I help her out? She would be most grateful and would recompense me when we meet in St Petersburg at Easter. Of course, I could help her out! And I send her £50 forthwith via Western Union. There is email silence for a few days, until she replies, thanking me for the £50, but telling me not to travel to St Petersburg as she will not be there to meet me. I've been scammed! Not the best introduction to international dating, but then, I had been naïve.

*

Somewhat surprisingly, a few of the *Eurocontact* ads are from Russian ladies who live in the UK, either temporarily or permanently. So I contact Julia who is in temporary residence in London with her sister, a UK citizen. Julia is from Belarus. When we meet, she's slim and attractive and smartly dressed with a white blouse and bright red trousers. It's a long time since I'd visited London and I'm more than happy to take her, at her request, to the Greenwich Observatory, where we stand astride the Meridian Line. We're getting on really well and after lunch, we link arms as we stroll through St James' Park in the warm Easter sun. We're relaxing on a park bench when, out of the blue, she asks: "So Jamie, how many lovers have you had?"

I'm surprised by her question and hope that she might want to join the list! After a quick count-up: "About 20, give or take one or two. How about you?"

I can see it's the wrong answer as she immediately unhooks her arm and moves to the far end of the bench, visibly shocked.

"Only one! My former husband before we divorced last year."

I've been honest—and naïve—again, and thereafter the date is difficult. Seeing no prospects for the future, we part at St James' Park tube station. Much to my surprise, she gives me a deep and lingering kiss—as if apologising for having raised such a delicate matter so soon. I curse myself for having been far too honest, and I'm left to wonder what might have been.

*

Next, I decide to meet Tanya, who lives near Oxford. It's a long cross-country drive for me but I'm willing to travel far on the basis of her pretty face and sexy photo. We meet up outside St Hilda's College where she'd recently been studying as a mature student. She's rather quiet and not as interesting as Julia—but not as inquisitive either! I sense some sexual tension, so I'm back the following weekend, where she takes me to the flat that she shares with another Russian lady, although she's away for the weekend. After returning from lunch, there's just the two of us in the kitchen getting coffee, when simultaneously we make for each other and start to kiss; before you can say *perestroika!*, we're making love on the living room carpet. After we've finished and with the sexual tension dissipated, I invite her to Grantham the following weekend, which she gladly accepts. At last! I seem to be getting somewhere with a Russian lady!

I meet her at the station, but immediately sense that something is different, but I don't know what. Perhaps she's nervous being with a strange man in a strange town. She stays overnight, although this time the love-making is perfunctory rather than passionate. The following morning, we go for a walk along the towpath of the derelict Grantham canal—but she's striding ahead of me in a world of her own. I can't work her out. What's going on?

After about twenty minutes, she stops and turns, and waits for me to catch up.

"Jamie, listen to me! Will you marry me? I need you to marry me! Please!"

I'm shocked and dumbfounded and just stare at her, trying to make some sense of it all.

"Tanya, we barely know each other. And you've been a bit strange this weekend. It's crazy to talk about marriage so soon! Why do you want to marry me anyway?"

There's a long pause as I await her reply as a blackbird sings sweetly in the hedgerow.

"Because I want to stay in the UK! My student visa ran out six months ago, and they'll come and deport me. I know they will. I've had a letter from

273

immigration. But if you marry me, I'll be allowed to stay and become a British citizen!"

I'm not pleased that she wants to use me in this way, and I tell her that it's completely out of the question. We return to my place where she gathers her things and I put her on the next train home. I'm disillusioned by my skirmishes with Russian women and their so-called 'traditional values'.

So I decide there will be no more skirmishes, just a full-scale adventure—to Russia itself!

2. St Petersburg

At the bus-stop in Nevsky Prospect, Svetlana explains: "Jamie, I had to kiss
you passionately in case the KGB were watching!"
That's about the craziest excuse I've ever heard for a snog and a fumble!

*

As well as buying the *Eurocontact* magazine, I also join *Introductions to Moscow*, a small family company that helps guys like me meet Russian ladies who are seeking partners from western Europe. They provide videos that contain photographs and basic information about their Russian lady clients. They also help with travel and visa arrangements and they have agents in both Moscow and St Petersburg who can meet men when they arrive and help arrange personal meetings with the Russian ladies.

I'm really interested in visiting St Petersburg because of its fascinating political and military history, especially the Bolshevik revolution of 1917 and the horrendous 900-day siege by the Nazis during the Second World War, in which 670,000 died, many from starvation.

*

For my 10-day August visit to St Petersburg, I devise a cunning plan! I will try to arrange dates with eight Russian ladies, one for each of the days I'm in the city, using the services of *Eurocontact* and *Introductions to Moscow*. I will ask each one to be my tour guide for the day around the city and in return, we'll have a meal together in a quality restaurant at my expense. If anything further develops, then that will be a bonus. Travel, culture, companionship and the possibility of romance, all packed into 10 days. It's a great plan! What can possibly go wrong?

From then on, I busy myself writing letters to suitable ladies in St Petersburg and reading their replies as they arrive some weeks later. Of all the ladies I'm in contact with, two stand out—Sveta (Svetlana) and Natasha. Sveta, I notice, has advertised in both the *Eurocontact* magazine and in the videos, so she must be keen—or desperate! Early on, she sends me her email address, so we communicate regularly and occasionally talk on the phone. As for Natasha, I see her photos and details in one of the videos. Of the hundreds of ladies in these videos all trying to look their best, Natasha stands out above them all. I'm immediately struck by her lovely figure, long dark hair, open face and friendly smile. Natasha doesn't have a computer so there's just one exchange of letters then one phone call a week before I'm due to travel. I'm already feeling enchanted but—"Jamie, I need to tell you this. My hair is different from the photos! I've gone blonde with some curls! I look more like Marilyn Monroe!"

I'm disappointed to hear that. I wanted to meet the beautiful lady in the video. I guess I'll just have to put up with Marilyn Monroe.

*

As I negotiate the terminals at Manchester then Frankfurt airports, I'm both excited and nervous. St Petersburg seems like an exotic world away—worlds apart from my life in Grantham—and the check-in queue is small compared to the madding crowds for warmer destinations. I travel with *Lufthansa* and on the comfortable leather seats, I finish a book about Lenin and test myself on my home-made flash-cards of Russian phrases. I've done my homework and I'm ready for anything!

Two agents from *Introductions to Moscow* greet me in Arrivals, then take me to *Hotel Moskva*, where they help me settle in and make a few phone calls for me to confirm arrangements for the next few days. The hotel is vast! The foyer is the size of a large ballroom, there are two restaurants and a café, and it takes five minutes to walk its entire length. The buffet breakfast is mind-boggling, arranged on linen-covered tables that seem to stretch a hundred yards along a ballroom balcony, while a pianist tinkles the ivories on the floor below. Being gastronomically conservative, I opt for a Russian version of an English breakfast—it's fabulous!

10 am in the foyer will be the regular meeting-time for my 'dates' or tour-guides, as I think of them. Over the next eight days, my guides take me to Peterhof Gardens by hydrofoil; to the *Aurora* Cruiser whose gunshot blank triggered the storming of the Winter Palace in 1917; to the *Peter and Paul*

Fortress; the famous *Hermitage* art gallery and museum; to *Nevsky Prospect*, the Oxford Street of St Petersburg; and to the River Neva and the nearby *Strelka* nightclub. There's so much to take in! In between my dates, I find time to visit the Alexander Nevsky Monastery just across the road from my hotel, where I run the gauntlet of two lines of beggars pleading for help.

Most claim to be Russian army veterans, each with a limb or two missing. I enter the church, where I observe with interest Orthodox worship taking place. It's so impressive that I make a second visit, this time taking enough roubles with me for each of the veterans.

*

I meet Sveta on my second day and we take a cruise around the city's canals, after which we walk by the River Neva, where I receive my first shock.

"Jamie, do you realise that the British Consulate won't allow a Russian lady to visit the UK without being married first?"

That was not the impression given to me by *Introductions to Moscow*—but I let her continue.

"But I'm lucky, as I already have a student visa with six months left. So I could come to visit you soon, to see where you live and meet your family and friends."

I think she's jumping the gun—just a bit! But I don't want to dissuade her too soon. We then visit the magnificent *Church on Spilled Blood*—the tourist symbol of St Petersburg—with its colourful onion-domes and striking azure-blue interior. We end the day in one of Hotel Moskva's restaurants before, approaching midnight, she departs for home. In the foyer, while waiting for her bus to arrive, she suddenly leans across and kisses me passionately on the lips, then grabs my crotch! I'm a bit shocked but I don't resist. She pulls me outside to the bus-stop, where she explains: "Jamie, I had to kiss you passionately in case the KGB were watching!"

It's the strangest reason I've ever been given for a kiss! However, I had read about the hotel's former notoriety for being a meeting place for criminals, the Russian mafia and the KGB. So Sveta explains that, as two single people, we could be thought to be dealing in contraband, but as a romantic couple, we would be ignored by any KGB present. I'm not at all convinced by her explanation but

I'm not complaining—for I haven't yet realised that Sveta has a cunning plan too!

I've nothing arranged for the following evening, so Sveta and I meet up in the same restaurant. After dinner, we move to my room and before long, she's stripping off and taking me to bed. She also tries a move on me, which she thinks will enhance my pleasure, but I tell her that her fingernails are too sharp, so she desists. We meet again on my final full day, in which she busies herself updating her visa and purchasing *Lufthansa* tickets to Manchester for her two-week visit to see me. Somewhat too late, I realise that I'm not really interested in Sveta— for I've been put off by her assertive nature, her manipulation of the situation and her dominating 'critical parent' personality. Her use of sex to dull my critical thinking has certainly worked a treat! And she maintains her treats up to and including my final evening before I leave St Petersburg.

In between my trysts with Sveta and my meeting with Natasha, I meet the other six ladies, including Tatiana who is very pretty and an Art teacher, but she is more interested in Rembrandt than me. Irina likes history, but she bores me stiff with her endless talk of Lenin's glorious revolution. Tanya takes me to a nightclub, where my eyes pop out at the other girls, but not at her.

*

On my penultimate night in the city, the lovely Natasha comes to meet me at Hotel Moskva. As she enters the foyer, heads turn—and it's not surprising! Natasha is tall and perfectly made-up with designer clothes—a short red jacket and an even shorter black skirt displaying a good length of her perfect legs. Her 'Marilyn' look is magnificent and I'm overjoyed to meet her. I'm stunned, so for a moment I hardly know where to look or what to say...

After a light meal and coffee, we take a walk to the nearby bridge over the River Neva, where we discuss our recent relationships at some length. She had recently been engaged to a guy from Finland who broke it off and subsequently returned to Helsinki. She's determined to get out dating again. I say nothing about Sveta. After a couple of hours, it's time for her to leave so we hug and say our farewells.

*

On the day of my departure from St Petersburg, the *Introductions* agents arrive in the foyer to assist my transfer to the airport—and Sveta turns up too! It's not what I was expecting or wanting. I need to speak to the agents discreetly, to get a message to Natasha that I'd like to meet her again. I manage to do this without Sveta knowing. In the car to the airport, they slip me a note without Sveta seeing. Natasha would also like to meet up again! In addition, the note contains her friend's email address for me to use.

Three weeks later, Sveta arrives in the UK, as she'd planned, and stays with me for two weeks. I take her to various places and she meets my mother, brother and best friend, Katie. Superficially, everything seems okay but in reality, it isn't. We share a bed again, but there's little interest on my part. The annoyances I felt in St Petersburg are still there so when the fortnight is over, I'm mightily relieved as I return her to the airport. I sense that she's disappointed but then, so am I.

Meanwhile, on my computer, I've already been exchanging emails with Natasha. She wants to meet again soon; would I like to spend a long weekend with her in Berlin?

3. Berlin Weekend

"I'm very sorry, Jamie. You're a very nice man but I cannot have sex with you."
It's honest—but it's not what I want to hear.

Two days after taking Sveta back to Manchester airport, terrorists hijack four airliners in the United States, flying two of them into the twin towers of the World Trade Centre, with a devastating loss of human life. It's 9/11 and everyone who witnessed the carnage on live TV, as I did, remembers exactly where they were and who they were with. President Kennedy, Princess Diana and now 9/11. The Cold War has ended, but the war on terror has begun. The world has changed.

As I board my early morning flight from Stansted to Berlin, I am more nervous than usual about the risks of flying, especially given the heavy October mist. I'm relieved when we touch down safely in Berlin despite the thick fog and low visibility.

*

The terminal building is relatively quiet and I find Natasha easily, who has already arrived from St Petersburg. She's still got the 'Marilyn' look, but somewhat understated compared with our first meeting. We catch a train to our hotel and I wait with interest as Natasha books us in at reception. She has booked just the one room—just as I'd hoped!

Having settled in, we decide on an open-top bus tour, as the sun filters through the vanishing mist. It's Natasha's first visit to the German capital, whereas I can recall my previous Bible-smuggling trip (2.3). How the city has changed since 1967! How *I* have changed since then! Natasha also seems to have changed in the short time since we met in St Petersburg—in fact, changed since her last email. She is standoffish and cool, which surprises and disappoints me.

I buy her some flowers but she won't accept them. I try to reach out to her, but she keeps pushing me away.

As we turn in early after a long day, Natasha changes in the en suite bathroom and slips into her bed without so much as a 'goodnight', let alone a goodnight kiss. I'm confused and it's a long, sleepless night. In the morning, over breakfast, nothing much has changed. Our day includes visits to the modern Kulterforum Museum and the Checkpoint Charlie Museum—but it feels that there's a wall between us, so I decide that before the day is over, I will tear down that wall if I possibly can—or at least challenge its existence.

Back at our hotel in late afternoon, we agree to take a nap before an evening meal in a city restaurant. Natasha surprises me by changing into her slinky nightwear. Then, rather than getting in bed, she sits on the bed reading a Russian newspaper. I decide it's time to act and, in my T-shirt and shorts, I sit on her bed and ask her what's the matter.

"I'm very sorry, Jamie. You're a very nice man but I cannot have sex with you. I told my former Finnish boyfriend I was meeting you and he said he wants to see me again—and I don't know what to do or what to think."

She sounds honest enough—but it's not what I want to hear! I need some time to process it all, so I excuse myself to use the bathroom, where I go for a think. While I'm there, I notice that the zip on Natasha's vanity bag is half-undone. I'm curious so I open the zip a little further and see an unopened box of condoms—curiouser and curiouser! I'm aware that I need to stay calm and try to be sympathetic towards her situation. There's nothing to be gained by being otherwise.

*

I return to sit on her bed and it looks as though she's been crying. We discuss her confusions at some length, which she seems to appreciate.

"Jamie, you're so understanding—unlike my Finnish boyfriend. Please hold me!"

She puts her paper on the floor and we hug. Before I know it, she's wrapping her leg around mine and tugging at my T-shirt, which she removes. For the first time, we enjoy warm eye contact and we start to kiss. I gently slip her camisole straps from off her shoulders, then lift it up and over her head, revealing her full and beautiful breasts. I don't know what to do first—but Natasha makes it clear that she wants to see some action, as she stretches back and invites me to remove her silk shorts and miniscule thong. I can now admire her wonderful naked body from head to toe; even Marilyn Monroe couldn't have looked any better than this!

Before long, Natasha nips into the bathroom to fetch her condoms, which we put to good use, before we sleep together naked and fall fast asleep. Hours later, I go in search of food and drink and return with a Chinese takeaway and two bottles of wine. It's the best evening meal in bed I've ever had! We push the beds together and spend the next three nights in each other's arms. Everything has changed between us. The wall has come down!

The next two days are as delightful as the previous two had been difficult. We have photos taken together, we visit the Europa centre for lunch and then admire the splendid blue and gold interior of the Kaiser Wilhelm Church, which I clearly remember from my previous visit. I have to smile when I compare the nature of my visit then with my visit now. Then, a Wall had just gone up. Now, a different type of wall has just come down! There's no more talk of Natasha's ex-boyfriend, just talk about our next opportunity to meet and the possibility of her visiting me in the UK. For our last two evenings, we dine in the hotel restaurant, then make a happy retreat to bed—though not to sleep, at least for long. As we finally kiss goodbye at Berlin's Schonefeld Airport, I'm high on love with thoughts of where and when our next weekend will be.

*

Back home in Grantham, I immediately email Natasha, thanking her for a wonderful weekend with suggestions about where we might meet next but I receive no reply. I'm concerned, so the following day after school, I phone her. I can tell from her voice that the excitement has gone—and I fear the worst. Once again she is honest, and once again she tells me what I don't want to hear: "Jamie, thank you for a lovely weekend, you are such a nice man. But when I returned, my Finnish boyfriend was waiting to meet me off the plane. He wants us to get back together and I've realised that's what I want too. I'm very sorry."

I can hardly believe my ears! I don't know whether to laugh or cry. I feel like crying, but the tears won't come. At least I can smile about those beautiful, blissful evenings! I'm so pleased that I'd had the maturity to stay in my 'Adult', keep calm and carry on…with Marilyn Monroe!

*

I come to view my Berlin weekend as a mixed blessing, and I wonder what to do next. In fact, I return to St Petersburg the following Easter, but it isn't as interesting or as much fun as my first trip. I don't really connect with any of my 'dates'—and I'm forced to admit that my Russian adventure has not delivered what I was hoping it would provide.

But then, not all revolutions are successful so perhaps *my* Russian Revolution is over too.

4. A Date in Kiev
December 2003

We leave the restaurant as snow is falling thick and fast around us. Anna holds on tightly to me as we turn into Victory Park and head back to the hotel. We've only just met, but it feels there's a connection between us already. So, as huge snowflakes continue to fall, I'm walking in a winter wonderland! However, I've been in similar situations before so it could be just a winter's tale that blows itself out by morning, or melts away with the first signs of spring.

*

After the second trip to St Petersburg, my cultural revolution continued apace but I'd more or less given up on the 'Russian revolution'. I was still keen to travel, to date and to mate. So, in the next eighteen months, I spent a long weekend in Stockholm, enjoyed two trips to Holland, a dance holiday in Barcelona and a long weekend in Bucharest. The trips were culturally diverse and always interesting: from Gaudi's amazing buildings in Barcelona and the gigantic Palace of Parliament in Bucharest to the red light district in Amsterdam. I've danced on the beaches in Barcelona, re-enacted the battle of *The Bridge Too Far* at Arnhem, smoked cannabis with Ed in Amsterdam and stood in *Piata Revolutiei* in Bucharest, where the dictator Ceaucescu had given his last speech before being captured and shot.

There had been a bit of dating but unfortunately no mating, and a long-term partner was as remote a prospect as ever. Whilst culturally I was on a high, emotionally I was slipping into another low mood and I only survived my dance-holiday in Barcelona through another course of anti-depressants. After my October trip to Bucharest, I resigned myself to another month of virtual dating through the recently discovered *Friendfinder* website. It was through this that I eventually receive a full and friendly reply from Anna in Kiev, whose good looks (I had assumed) had put her out of my reach.

A flurry of emails and photos pass between us before Anna invites me to visit her and her mother in Kiev—so this invitation sounds promising. I fly out from Stansted on a Friday evening in mid-December, spend the night in the Transit centre at Frankfurt airport and, after a lengthy shower and first-class breakfast, make my way to the *Lufthansa* flight to Kiev.

Anna, tall, blonde and smiling, is there to greet me at the bitterly cold airport, then helps me settle into my gloomy Soviet-era hotel, where she is staying too, although in a different room. By the time we walk through Victory Park to the city centre, a few snowflakes are falling and I notice that with her fur hat and coat and furry boots, she is much better protected against a central European winter than me. We hold each other close to keep warm as she shows me around the city-sights, before taking me to the restaurant where she has booked a table. It's a busy Saturday night in the restaurant, where Anna and I are soon seated and continue to talk nonstop. I've already made up my mind—I want to see her again. After the meal is over, I feel it's time to find out what Anna is thinking about me. Without hesitation, she confides to me in her excellent English: "I enjoy your company too and we have a lot in common—so I'd like to meet you again!"

*

By the time we leave the restaurant, the snow is several feet thick. The restaurant walls are high, with windows only at the top, so we were unaware of the severity of the snowfall outside. As we plough our way back through the park, the wind whips up the snow and we cling on tightly to each other, ending up at the hotel looking like abominable snowmen! When I eventually hit the pillow, I'm soon asleep, knowing that after this trip ends, we'll be meeting again in the New Year.

In the morning, we breakfast together in the sixth-floor restaurant. Outside, it's dismal, grey and misty and nothing moves. Anna soon brightens the gloom by presenting me with a birthday gift—two glass swans joined at the neck on a heart-shaped base, bearing two glass rings. It's a touching gesture, if a bit presumptive—but I'm not complaining. After breakfast, Anna takes me to her flat to meet her mother who is very welcoming. She only found out the previous month that Anna was dating men outside Ukraine, so it cannot be easy for her—but outwardly, she shows no sign of resentment.

After coffee and Ukrainian delicacies with her mother, we travel by taxi to Independence Square, where we spend an hour or so before leaving for the airport. It's there, while I'm waiting to check in, that we share our first real kiss—long, warm and passionate despite the public gaze.

*

Once aboard the early afternoon flight, I start to relax and recover from my 24-hour whirlwind visit to Kiev. I'm looking forward to another visit in January, although the thought crosses my mind that Anna could just be a well-rehearsed actress in search of a British passport and citizenship through marriage. It's with mixed feelings then that I return home to Grantham, to finish off some essay-marking and get ready for Monday morning lessons. But at least the trip had seemed more productive than usual and had not been another long-distance disaster.

My January trip to Kiev feels more relaxed and reassuring, although again it's only a 24-hour flying visit. This time, Anna arranges a more welcoming and friendly hotel and we share a room, though not a bed. We agree that we need to spend more time together, to get to know each other better than these whirlwind visits will allow. We discuss various options and decide that a week in Cyprus during my February half-term would be the best arrangement. Anna has been before, and it's popular with Russian-speaking tourists. It's also a haven for British tourists and expats because of its former British influence and its two permanent RAF bases.

Back at Anna's apartment, we make our plans for some Cypriot winter warmth, which is now only a month away. By the time February arrives, a lot of questions are building up in my mind that I need to ask Anna. And I expect that in Cyprus, she will be curious about me as well.

5. Curious in Cyprus

Just as we were leaving the hotel, we had our first disagreement: "You can't
go out like that—wearing blue and red. It's not stylish!"
"It might not be stylish in Russia, but we're not in Russia now. And in Britain,
we can wear what we want, without the need for the fashion police!"
"I don't live in Russia!" Anna reminds me. "I live in Ukraine!"

*

Having arrived in Cyprus and settled in at the Holiday Inn in Limassol, this was the first time that Anna and I had stepped out on foreign soil together—and straight into our first tiff. But it was quickly forgotten. This was to be a 'make or break' week for us as I could not afford a £500 trip to Kiev every month to see Anna for just 24 hours. I arrive with a whole stack of questions to put to her, to see if we have enough common ground for a long-term future together—or not.

Questions such as:

- Was Anna's mother really accepting of her only child leaving her and leaving Ukraine?
- What did her father think? (Her parents had divorced some years previously.)
- Why had she split up from her former husband?
- What did Anna know about, and expect from, life in the UK?
- Was religion important to her?
- How important was marriage to her?
- How important was sex?
- Did she want children?
- Did she want to travel more widely?
- Would she like to learn to dance?

During the first few days, I manage to put these questions to her and she has a few for me too.

In virtually all cases, her attitude and outlook seem to match my own, although her father is not happy about her moving away and so refuses to meet me. We do have some differences of interest—notably Anna's routine of meditation before breakfast and each evening. It reminds me of all those hours I had spent in prayer as an evangelical Christian and Anglican minister. I hope she won't try to convert me to meditation, as she'd be wasting her time! During her hour-long morning meditation, I do some background reading about Greek philosophy—for I had recently been told at school to prepare for 'A' level philosophy of religion classes later on in the year (5.9). So while Anna meditates, I have time to read. It's a good arrangement—although deeply symbolic of our differences, which (of course) we do not recognise at the time.

As for sex and marriage, we share the same bed from our first evening together and our love-making is passionate and mutually satisfying. We spot some exotic and skimpy lingerie on one of our shopping trips, which Anna is keen to buy for some nocturnal fun later on. We seem to be on the same, exciting page!

Marriage is a trickier issue for me. I'm conflicted—because of Maggie's prior warning that a partner's over-availability might reduce my sexual interest. On the other hand, I really want some stability—so marriage will surely provide that. Anna has no such reservations about marrying, even though she's been married—and divorced—already. But she assures me, on the basis of some friends' experiences, that the British Embassy in Kiev will not grant her a UK Settlement visa unless we are married first. This puts a lot of pressure on me as I'm not convinced about the wisdom of being married at all! And I'm only too aware of the old adage: *marry in haste, repent at leisure!*

Nevertheless, as the week progresses, I feel increasingly drawn to Anna—and I cannot imagine spending the future without her, or with seeing her for only one day a month. She's the beautiful young lady that I've been searching for, for many a long year—am I going to throw this opportunity away just because we need to get married sooner than I expected? If Anna is right for me, then why worry? On the Thursday morning, as we are walking in the glorious sunshine by the Fort at Paphos harbour, I make up my mind—but say nothing to Anna.

*

288

We enjoy Paphos so much that we agree to stay for a few more hours so that I can explore the Fort area and Anna can do some clothes shopping. While we're apart, I phone the hotel and arrange to upgrade our room from inland-facing to a sea-view with a balcony. After our return and a jacuzzi together, I lead Anna to our new room overlooking the Mediterranean. She's impressed! At my request, there is also champagne and flowers waiting for us on the balcony and, while the sun is setting, I propose to her. Unfortunately, I wrap up my proposal with various conditional clauses, such as her mother's approval, and Anna is not happy about this.

"Just ask me to marry you! With no ifs and no buts!"

"Okay, will you marry me?"

"Yes! Of course I will!"

Events move swiftly thereafter and the next morning, we're off to a jeweller's in Limassol to select two engagement rings, although we decide to leave the official engagement to my March visit to Kiev. We discuss possible wedding locations. It can't be in the UK without a visa and Anna doesn't want Kiev, as it's not romantic and will only remind her of her first unhappy marriage.

We're in a café when we see a brochure that advertises weddings in Cyprus—and the idea immediately appeals! We really like Paphos, so we head back to the Town Hall to see if they have a summer vacancy. They haven't—they are booked up throughout the summer. However, they do have one vacancy in early April—are we interested? We think about it for two seconds then look at each other. "Yes please, we'll take it!" And we spend the rest of the day in a lazy, loved-up haze by the bright, bobbing boats in Paphos harbour.

*

It's only on the plane back to Stansted that I start to reflect upon what I've just done.

I've met a complete stranger on the Internet, who is from the other side of Europe.

On our first date, I meet her mother.

At the end of our third date, I propose, and our fifth date will be our wedding day!

But what if both our mothers became set against it?

Or Anna doesn't like the UK once she's arrived?

Or gets cold feet, and never makes it across the English Channel?

Or if the excitement of our overseas love affair turns into a cultural conflict?

Or mismatched personalities emerge from behind well-adapted romantic exteriors?

*

The possibilities for disaster seem endless if I stop to think about it. It's one thing having a spirited 'free child' and taking the odd risk. But throwing myself headlong into an unknown, uncertain, overseas marriage so quickly is surely bordering on the insane?

6. Stick or Twist?

There's an unpleasant twist to our first visit to the British Embassy in Kiev. Even if we get married, there's still no guarantee that Anna will be granted a Settlement visa for the UK. We could get married—but Anna could still be stuck in Kiev and I'd be stuck in Grantham! We are told that most applications are approved after about two months, but some are rejected. When we ask why some are rejected, they refuse to tell us.

Perhaps they reject couples who rush into marriage on their fifth date! I think to myself. So we leave the embassy downhearted—despite having gained some useful information about the documentation needed for the visa application, such as copies of emails between us, itemised phone bills, recent photos and identification documents. About a dozen types of items in all.

*

I'm back in Kiev in March for a long weekend—to get engaged and to plan for an April wedding! We discuss a multitude of details about our wedding arrangements; we confirm the time and date with Paphos Town Hall; we book hotels in Larnaca and Paphos; and decide that I will travel to and from Kiev at both ends of the fortnight in Cyprus. We go ahead and book the necessary flights. It's getting expensive: I shall need a bank loan! Back in Grantham, I see the bank manager and it's all arranged. However, I worry about Anna's mother. Outwardly, she seems pleased for us but I've no idea what she's really thinking beneath her demure exterior. I can only speak a few Russian phrases and she knows no English, so there's no direct communication.

*

On April Fool's Day, Anna and I meet in the Transit centre at Frankfurt-Main airport. It's exciting! But am I being an April fool? We fly off to Larnaca, where we stay for a few days and get suited and booted in white, with light blue shirts, a white tie for me and flowers for Anna—as well as the two wedding rings, of course. We then drive to Paphos to stay in a 5-star hotel for five nights. The wedding at the Town Hall goes, more or less, without a hitch. The only problem is the bumbling secretary, who continues to shuffle papers noisily throughout the ceremony and then makes a complete hash of the marriage certificate, which we only notice in the taxi back to the hotel. So we have to return to the Town Hall to get all the mistakes corrected. A bonus, however, is that as we depart for the second time, we ask a professional photographer (who is there for the next wedding) to take some photos with our own cameras—and so end up with perfect wedding photos, for free!

After a few days in Paphos to relax in the harbour area once more, we head off to Nicosia to get our marriage formally ratified, thereby securing another document necessary for Anna's settlement visa. We also fit in a day trip to Agia Napa, for a lovely swim in its clear warm waters. Then finally, a return flight from Larnaca to Kiev—and to the British Embassy with Anna's visa application.

We wait nervously at the embassy for Anna to be called for her hour-long interview—her opportunity to convince the officials that we are a genuine couple. She takes the four volumes of documentation that I have been preparing over the past two months. We hope it will be adequate. After that, it's a two-month wait while her application is processed and approved—or rejected.

The following morning, Anna gets an unexpected phone call from the British Embassy. They want to see her again as soon as possible about her application. We are full of foreboding and fear the worst, as Anna is called into the interview room. But she appears a few minutes later with a huge smile across her face: the Settlement visa has already been approved—and with immediate effect! We can hardly believe it! Anna was told that she had interviewed very well, and that my documentation was the best they had ever seen—so it was an easy decision for them to approve it.

Scarcely daring to believe our luck, we immediately make plans for Anna to make an initial week-long visit to the UK during my summer half-term and then return to Kiev to work off her notice at the restaurant where she works and say goodbye to her mother and her friends. She would then return to the UK—for good—at the end of July. That's the plan, so it's fingers crossed!

*

I'm overjoyed to welcome Anna at Stansted and introduce her to my hometown, my mother, brother and friends. Without exception, they all find her charming and look forward to seeing her in the UK on a permanent basis. I take her on a whistle-stop tour of London, Oxford and Stonehenge, all of which impress her a great deal. The week flies quickly by and before we know it, we're back at the airport—and Anna is looking tearful.

"Jamie, I love you very much. But I'm so worried about leaving my mother alone in Kiev. I'm all she has and she was upset before I left for this visit. I don't know what to do. I don't want to leave her alone—yet I want to have my own life too."

I'm shocked by what Anna is saying, although I can understand her close attachment to her mother.

We are both struggling to hold back tears as, after a final hug, Anna leaves for the Gate. As she disappears with a wave, questions surge through my head:

Will I ever see her again?
Am I going to end up with a long-distance marriage?
Will she stick with me and our future?
Or will she return to the life she knows with her mum?
Will she stick—or will she twist?

7. The Unforgettable Morning
August 2004

Anna got up, wrapped a large towel around herself, then drew back the curtains to enjoy the sea view. That was the moment when I realised—that our fledgling marriage could be over by the end of the day!

*

Due to the complex arrangements for our marriage in Cyprus and for obtaining Anna's Settlement visa, we decided to delay a proper honeymoon until after Anna had arrived in Britain on a permanent basis, at the end of July. Right up to the moment that she texted me from the plane, I was anxious and unsure if she would finally make it—and overjoyed when she finally appeared through the sliding door in Arrivals! Now we could really set out on our life together!

Before departing for our honeymoon, we decide to order a new bed, which will be delivered immediately upon our return. After visiting a number of showrooms, Anna eventually decides on the one she wants—a super king-size. I ask her why she is so set on this particular bed, considering it will hardly fit into our bedroom.

"Because it's the biggest one we've seen, and I've lots of sexy ideas that we'll need a bit of space for!"

I don't need further convincing—can there be any luckier man in the world than me? What more could I want than a beautiful new wife who wants to experiment with her sexuality with me! I can't wait for the new bed to arrive, and to find out exactly what ideas she has in mind! So we set off to the south coast, full of anticipation and with great expectations of married life together.

*

The first places we visit are Salisbury and Winchester where we stay for a couple of nights each.

Then on to the coast: to Poole Harbour, Sandbanks, Christchurch and the New Forest. At our sea-view hotel in Christchurch, Anna gets out of bed one morning, wraps a large towel around herself, then draws back the curtains to enjoy the sea view. As she stands there, looking so beautiful, I suddenly blurt out: "Oh my God! It's happened again! I can't believe it!"

But believe it I do.

Anna turns around to ask me what's the matter.

"I'm very sorry, but I don't really fancy you anymore! This has happened before and I was hoping it wouldn't happen again—but it has."

Anna can't make any sense of my words, as sex has been great between us, from our second meeting in Kiev until now—it's just ridiculous to think otherwise. However, deep down, I know what has just happened in my brain and why. So I try to explain:

"Everything was fine while our relationship was uncertain and unsettled. Even after we'd got married, there were doubts about the visa, your mother and whether you would actually make it to the UK to live with me permanently. While we were flying about and everything was 'up in the air', my sexual response was strong—as you know.

"But now that you are fully available for me—living together and with your plans for the super king-size bed—I've lost my desire and I don't see it coming back."

I can see that Anna is still struggling to grasp what I'm trying to say, so I continue: "It was when I woke up this morning and saw you at the window—I saw you as beautiful, lovely and gorgeous—but I just didn't *feel* anything, either down below or in my head. It was just like a switch being turned off. Being overloaded with your availability is literally a 'turn-off'. I'm very, very sorry. I knew this was a possibility but I couldn't be certain. Maggie was right—though I hoped I would prove her wrong.

"That's why I didn't want to get married in the first place, if you remember. I thought that just living together, and remaining unmarried, would keep the uncertainty, and the sex, alive."

Anna's got questions:

"But if this is true, then *why*—I don't understand."

I try to explain: "When I was just twelve months old, my mother received some devastating news that resulted in her being clinically depressed for a long time (1.1). This meant that when I wanted a cuddle or affection from her, I rarely got it and as a result, I became anxious.

"Sometimes I received affection, sometimes I didn't, but I could never tell which it would be. Therefore, my developing brain started to associate love and affection with uncertainty and anxiety, but never with availability and unconditional love. My brain seems to be hard-wired as a result of this repeated experience when it was still developing.

"The anxiety of a new or uncertain relationship gets me really interested— and I get turned on. But when someone, like yourself, offers me love and affection all the time and without any conditions, my brain can't process it, because it's not wired that way. It's a bugger!"

Anna looks thoughtful: "It all sounds very Freudian to me."

"Yes, it does, but it's not. It's known as 'maternal deprivation'. It was John Bowlby who first realised that if an infant is denied consistent emotional warmth and affection in those crucial early years, its effects can be damaging and long-lasting, even for a lifetime. It's called Attachment Theory."

"We'll talk more later. Let's go for breakfast."

8. Beating the Blues I

Breakfast is consumed solemnly and thoughtfully, with minimum conversation. We are clearly both shaken by what's just happened and I'm wondering if Anna will be packing her bags and heading back to Kiev before the day is out...

However, once back in our room, we declare our love for each other and our commitment to the relationship, whatever difficulties might lie in the way. This is marriage—but not as we expected! We can still share our love and affection for each other and enjoy skin-to-skin contact. It's just that 'normal' sex appears to be off the menu, judging from my past—and now present—experience.

Over the next few months, we discuss ways by which we might overcome my loss of sexual functioning within the marriage. The most obvious is for Anna to appear less 'available'—to play 'hard to get'. We try this for a while, but it feels very false and my brain is not taken in by it. Another possibility is to role-play ourselves as various characters who are strangers—scenes in which, for example, Anna dresses up provocatively as if in a nightclub, while I attempt to chat her up and eventually seduce her. It sounds great in theory but neither of us can get into role without laughing and giving the game away—and my brain gives our performances only a one-star rating.

After a few years together, with affection but not sex, I suggest a more radical idea—that Anna rent a flat on the other side of town and we date, like boyfriend and girlfriend. That might do the trick. I also suggest the possibility that, in this arrangement, we could also take other partners—an open marriage. *That* would surely trigger my brain and body into a high state of jealousy, anxiety and desire. But it's a high-risk strategy and we both decide it's not what either of us really wants. We want our lives to be lived together, not apart, and not with other people. And in her newly adopted country, it's very important to Anna that she feels more secure, not less. Eventually, we come to accept that the situation appears unresolvable. We continue to cuddle and be affectionate, but sharing a common bed without sex is starting to feel awkward so we agree to sleep in separate rooms.

Meanwhile, there are other practical problems for us to deal with—primarily concerning employment for Anna. It seems that she can't get a job without a National Insurance number, and she can't obtain a National Insurance number without a job! It's a strange system! Thankfully, a local ladies' clothes shop agrees to employ Anna on the basis of her proof of identity, her settlement visa and our marriage certificate. Anna doesn't enjoy the job, but she gets a National Insurance number so progress is made. Within a year, she finds more suitable employment working in the International Department at a local college. So her employment problems are getting resolved.

One condition of her new employment is that she has to upgrade her educational qualifications, as her three-year degree in English Literature at the University of Kiev is not recognised by UK authorities! We both feel piqued at this disregard of her existing qualifications, but she has to comply. So Anna attends evening classes for GCSE-equivalent exams in English and Maths, and I ferry her there and back and help her with her study—not that she needs much help as she's a fast learner. Unsurprisingly, but with great relief, she passes both exams with top grades!

Next, Anna plans to learn to drive and own her own car. She's also keen to become a British citizen as soon as it is possible. Now in full-time employment, she can afford to pay for her own driving lessons, and I agree to pay half towards a car after she passes her test. She passes the theory exam easily and takes her driving test after a minimum number of lessons, passing the first time! One benefit of this is that she can now drive herself to her Sunday morning meditation meetings in Nottingham—a task that I had happily undertaken for her first four years.

By now, the lack of sex in our marriage seems a relatively minor issue. It's Project Anna that is sustaining and fulfilling our marriage with all of her achievements.

It seems that we are beating the blues.

Before long, Anna is busy attending British citizenship meetings in Lincoln and preparing for the exams. Having now lived in the UK for over three years, and with a thorough study of the government-issued textbooks, she passes the exams with ease and becomes a British citizen in 2008 at a ceremony in Lincoln City Hall.

Anna has, by now, also learned to dance modern jive so our social life is improving too, as we attend a couple of dance-nights per week, usually together, but occasionally on our own. My life has been so wrapped up in Anna's for the past four years that I'm starting to feel a loss of my own sense of self. So when I go to a dance by myself, I enjoy the freedom—and allow myself a little flirtation.

At school, my work is going from strength to strength. My sixth-form students are continuing to achieve good AS and A2 results in sociology and psychology, and more students are applying to take these subjects each year. Of particular significance, however, are the results of the first group of philosophy of religion students that completed both AS and A2 exams in 2007 (5.9). It's not only the results that are gratifying. It's also the way they'd all helped and supported each other, the more able helping the less able—and with all beliefs in the group being respected as well as debated: Christian, Muslim, agnostic and atheist. I feel much valued by their generous comments in their joint 'thank you' card, as well as the compliment paid to me by some Muslim girls: "Sir, the textbooks are good, but you explain things so much better and you always give us some new ideas to think about!"

It seems that Project sixth-form teaching is helping me beat my own particular blues.

9. Beating the Blues II
"Can we do it? Yes, we can!"

Barack Obama: 2008

During the first part of our marriage, two key 'projects' helped distract Anna and myself from the vulnerability of a sexless relationship: Project Anna and Project sixth-form teaching. There was also a third element of mutual interest that had been present from our first correspondence and was integral to our developing relationship: Project international travel. Travel had been a key feature of my 'cultural revolution' (6.7-8) and it was important to Anna too, with her limited opportunities thus far, to see the world. Thus, international travel and its planning was less of a specific project and more the life-giving bloodstream for our relationship.

*

For our first five years, we opt for the warmer and sunnier climes of southern Europe: two trips to Cyprus in the year we get married, then Crete and Santorini, Malta, Granada in southern Spain and back again to Cyprus for our fifth wedding anniversary. Once Anna had received her British passport, these and other trips become much easier as she doesn't need to apply for special travel visas. So we head off for short breaks to various capital cities: Paris, Amsterdam, Bern and Madrid. We have a fortnight planned for Vienna and Salzburg but we have to cancel as Anna's elderly mother becomes seriously ill, so Anna returns to Kiev to nurse her. Months later, Anna returns to Kiev again to oversee her funeral arrangements. The following year, we're planning a trip to Singapore when project house extension becomes more important and we decide to cancel in order to oversee the building work.

*

My house isn't really big enough for the two of us, and we would like to add a downstairs study and guest-room. So we apply for a bank loan, an architect is called in and plans are made for a single-storey extension to the side of the house. However, the day before the diggers are due to arrive, our builders inform us that the job can't be done due to the presence of a drain that would require foundations twice as deep and would double the cost. Disappointed by the news, I threaten legal action against the architect, but he settles outside court. We then decide to use the bank loan for the renovation of the whole house, primarily a new kitchen and bathroom—but no wall or room is left untouched. Anna has a fitted wardrobe in her bedroom for her extensive clothes collection, and I have new shelves for my extensive book collection and a new computer to assist my increasing workload of reading, preparation and marking.

Almost without noticing, my sixth-form work is becoming more and more important, day by day, lesson by lesson. With almost a hundred students depending on quality lessons for their exam success, there's no let up. Sunday becomes virtually another working day for me, with my main weekend treat being a Saturday trip to *Waterstones* for the latest book on Nietzsche, Postmodernism or Lifespan psychology. There are compensations however—not only do I enjoy the intellectual adventure, but I enjoy seeing the students similarly engaged. For, despite the hard work required of them, they are always chirpy and full of good humour and bright ideas.

"Hi sir! What are we doing today?" is their familiar greeting on the corridor before each lesson.

"Hard work with a smile!" is my familiar answer. Our work *is* hard—but it's also a buzz!

*

Having missed out on Singapore and having already visited many European destinations, Anna and I decide on a new travel adventure—the USA! Due to a shortage of funds, our first visit is relatively short and cheap—to Orlando, Florida, during my October half-term holiday. We plan to visit selected Disneyland parks and the Kennedy Space Centre at Cape Canaveral. We prepare by watching the first few episodes of *Stephen Fry in America* [123] and by obtaining the relevant travel guides for what lies ahead, including possible trips to Orlando itself and the Everglades.

However, during a coffee break en route to the Kennedy Space Centre, I spot in a local newspaper that Barack Obama has a pre-election rally that evening in Kissimmee, just ten miles from our hotel on International Drive. We decide that we want to go, so the coach driver phones for a taxi to pick us up on our way back to Orlando. The queue at the stadium is long and without street lighting, but we manage to shuffle into the line unnoticed—and we leave our day-bags in a police car as no bags are allowed inside the stadium. We also get a bonus—Bill Clinton is there, and he gets a rapturous reception from the majority black and mixed-race crowd—something the British media never reports on. After Clinton's excellent warm-up act, Barack Obama appears and the crowd goes wild—as they can hardly believe that a black guy *might* be America's next President—you can see the anxiety etched on their faces. "Can we do it?" asks Obama. "Yes, we can!" comes their overwhelming response! And of course, six days later, they did. It was the high spot of our holiday to be part of that crowd.

*

Then, the following year, to mark my 60th birthday, Anna and I spend four days in New York, with our hotel just walking distance from Times Square and Broadway. We take in all the major sights and see Britney Spears in her *Circus* show in Madison Square Garden. She's looking and sounding good on this, her comeback tour after her recent and well-publicised meltdown and shaven head! The helicopter flight over Manhattan was breath-taking and provided our best memory. Project USA is well underway, with more trips to come.

Two years later, to celebrate Anna's 50th birthday, she suggests, by way of a change, a trip to Jordan: to visit the River Jordan itself and the ancient city of Petra, to swim in the Dead Sea and for her to cover herself in the lake's thick black mud! We also visit Amman, but our taxi-driver is so nervous that we expect either him, or us, to be hijacked by terrorists at any moment. But we outwit them all and survive!

Later that summer, as a pre-retirement adventure, we plan a coast-to-coast trip across America, using Amtrak's double-decker sleeper trains for transport. It's an excellent two-week trip, taking in Washington DC, Chicago, Santa Fe, the Grand Canyon and Los Angeles—and ending up on the Pacific beach at Santa Monica. In Washington, we visit the Kennedy graves, wave to Barack and Michelle in the White House and watch a live debate in Congress. In LA, we inspect Hollywood's 'Walk of Fame', before bidding farewell to Roy Orbison and Marilyn Monroe at their resting places in Westwood Village Memorial Park.

Of lesser fame is Calvin Kristoffersen, who sings Country and Blues on the local train down to the magnificent Grand Canyon. His songs remind me of an alternative America—the America of Bob Dylan and Johnny Cash. Once back home in the UK, I'm inspired to go and see Bob Dylan in concert, together with Ed. He opens with *Things Have Changed*—a rocky number, well known in the UK dance halls of modern jive.

But unbeknown to me, 'things' were also about to change in my life— changes that would rock my world and would send me spiralling downwards into the darkness once more.

10. Russian Revolution: Review
2001–2011

i.   All forms of 'dating', where one is essentially meeting a stranger, carry some level of risk irrespective of whether the date is met through a lonely hearts column or through *Tinder*. International dating through the Internet carries a much higher level of risk, not only through the uncertainties of foreign travel and unfamiliar cultures but emotionally, through the success or otherwise of the dating objectives, whatever they may be.

ii.   Through combining a genuine desire to travel and experience new cultures, with dating, I felt I was reducing the emotional risk. If the dates were unsuccessful, I always had the travel and cultural experience to make the adventure worthwhile. I felt therefore that I had a measure of emotional security built into my trips to St Petersburg and Berlin. It's true that while still in the UK, I had been lured into Elena's scam and into a potential crime by Tanya (7.1), but overall I started to feel that my 'cultural revolution' was providing me with a 'secure base' for my dating adventures. Perhaps it was part of the process of 'earning' myself a secure attachment (3.10).

iii. In St Petersburg itself, my relationship with Sveta was a mixed bag. The positives were sexual and immediate, but the negatives took a bit longer to work out: sex can have an inhibiting effect upon one's cognitive processes—and perhaps Sveta deliberately played on that: bed, wed, UK passport, bingo! Even while Sveta was rushing around and barking at officials about her visa and air tickets, I felt almost certain that her 'critical parent' personality was not for me and I should have stopped her in her tracks. But my counsellor, Maggie, had often warned me against judging dates too quickly, and so I held back. It was only during her stay with me in Grantham that I became aware that she was also too sexually available for my liking. Doubtless it was part of her cunning plan, but if so, it had spectacularly backfired. In any case, I soon realised that I just wasn't interested in her as a person—especially after she had complained about all the 'immigrants' she'd seen in Grantham and Nottingham, rather overlooking the fact that they were British citizens with roots in Commonwealth countries—whereas she was the real immigrant! A fact I was quick to point out to her.

iv.   My dates with Natasha in St Petersburg and Berlin (7.2-3) were the stuff of romantic novels—apart from the ending. But the journey en route to that ending was both enjoyable and unforgettable. Natasha had done the very opposite to Sveta, in that she had become emotionally distant then sexually unavailable. Though initially disappointed, I was hooked by the challenge to discover the reasons for her coolness. Then, after my sexual rejection, I was pleased that I got into my 'Adult' and 'Nurturing Parent' roles—when I could have so easily descended into my 'Child' and 'Critical Parent'. And I reaped the rewards of Natasha's appreciation of those particular transactions!

v.   However, if it is true that sex can make you forget things, then surely good sex can make you forget a lot of things—even a lot of important things! This is why I forgot virtually everything about Natasha's Finnish boyfriend: in my blissful state, he simply did not exist. Unfortunately for me, in the real world, he did.

vi.   If to marry someone on a fifth date is foolhardy, then to marry someone on a fifth *international* date is plain reckless. But reckless we were, which demonstrated that Anna and I had at least one thing in common— a very active 'Free Child' spirit. To that extent, we were a good match. With my experiences with Georgie (5.7) and Sveta to learn from, I could have interpreted Anna's enthusiasm for our relationship along similar lines, i.e., too available, and perhaps with an ulterior motive. But I didn't, partly because it was me and not Anna who initiated our first sexual encounter. In addition, there was no obvious neediness in Anna's character, unlike both Georgie and Sveta. To me she seemed securely attached, with a positive relationship with her mother. All this indicated that an early marriage was not necessarily doomed to failure—it *might* work out okay. In any case, even five years of dating in Kiev would not have shown us what marriage in the UK would be like.

vii.   I had, however, a couple of slight concerns—apart from the huge risks we were both taking! The first one is that part of me would have preferred to simply live together rather than get married, as marriage suggests complete and lifelong availability, both personal and sexual. On the other hand, I wanted the security of marriage—as all my previous relationships had failed for one reason or another. I wanted this one to last! So I was very conflicted about the issue. In the end, the decision was taken out of our hands as it became clear that according to the British Embassy, we *had* to get married if Anna was to have any chance of getting a Settlement visa to join me in the UK. As far as the British Embassy was concerned, there was no other way.

viii.   My second concern was that, over the four months between our first meeting and our marriage, Anna was completely reliable. If she said she would phone me at 10 am on a Sunday morning, then 10 am it would be. At no point did she demonstrate any uncertainty or unreliable behaviour. I could totally trust her. At a human level, this was very good for me and spared me from all manner of anxieties. There was no personal uncertainty about Anna. However, psychologically, it did feel rather strange that I didn't experience any 'butterflies in my stomach' about our developing relationship. Nor any 'separation-anxiety' when we were apart, as we often were. I realised that I needed *some* form of anxiety in the relationship to maintain my interest, both personal and sexual.

ix.   However, in the six months between our first meeting and Anna's arrival to live permanently in the UK, there was in fact, a great deal of *situational uncertainty* to maintain my anxiety levels. The very fact that we were flying hither and thither, getting flights, visas and a marriage arranged, plus concern about Anna's mother, meant that we were never free from anxiety and uncertainty. It was an exciting six months! Enough anxiety to keep my sexual interest high—and even getting married didn't dampen my ardour as there was still a great deal of situational turbulence—with the potential for things to go wrong—between our April marriage and Anna's final arrival in late July.

x.   It was only when Anna arrived in the UK on a permanent basis that things started to feel flat because: 1. There was no personal uncertainty about Anna. 2. We were married and living together—so no uncertainty there. 3. There was no longer any situational uncertainty anymore because things were no longer 'up in the air'—neither physically or psychologically.

xi.   It took my brain just a few days to register the new situation of nil uncertainty before 'The Unforgettable Morning' arrived.

xii.   It is typical of the desires and behaviour of those ambivalently attached to want something, or someone, very badly for a long period of time and then, when it arrives or is achieved, to reject it in one way or another. Such behaviour mirrors that of some children in Mary Ainsworth's *Strange Situation* experiment who, upon the return of their mother to the room, first seek her comfort, then push her away and wriggle until they are put down. Such children are ascribed an 'ambivalent' status by the researchers [124] and their behaviour reminds me of my own childhood.

xiii.   It is gratifying to know that, being ambivalently attached myself, I fit into the general pattern of anxious/ambivalent behaviour—although there are wide variations within this. For example: Gillath and Schachner (2006) found that "attachment anxiety was related to a preference for a long-term mating strategy, presumably because of a desire for reliable love, acceptance and protection." [125]. This was indeed the case with my own life-long search for a long-term partner.

xiv.   However, as Esther Perel writes: *No history has a more lasting effect on our adult loves than the one we write with our primary caregivers… The psychology of our desire often lies buried in the details of our childhood* [126]. She goes on to say that the *erotic blueprint…illustrates the irrationality of our desire…that what excites us most, often arises from our childhood hurts and frustrations* [127]. That is why I found the sexual rejection by Natasha more erotically exciting than the reliable availability of Anna because, in my brain, I have a hard-wired neuronal blueprint for such rejection from my mother—but no such blueprint to help me with Anna's available and reliable love.

xv.   Susan Kuchinskas explains in more detail: *In the first three years of life, the brain goes through a huge growth spurt, nearly tripling in size and forging billions of connections between neurons. Neural scripts, the habitual patterns of emotional response, begin to develop… At the same time, a use-it-or-lose-it process called neural pruning begins: while the parts of the brain that get more use become stronger, neurons that aren't used wither away.* [128]. Therefore, my lack of desire towards Anna on the Unforgettable Morning is due to my lack of neural connections that register available and reliable love. And that lack goes right back to the events of the Unforgettable Night (1.1) and its consequences for my child care over the next two years.

xvi.   The cameo with Natasha neatly illustrates, I believe, the relationship between hard-wired insecure attachment from infancy and earned security from adulthood. It was my hard-wired ambivalence that generated the erotic interest, being triggered by the situational uncertainty. But my cool and adult response of how to deal with the situation was, I believe, the consequence of earned security that had arisen from the secure base of my 'cultural revolution' (see *i* above).

xvii.   It is also worth noting that my knowledge of Attachment theory, and of myself, prevented the Unforgettable Morning from descending into a 'blame-game' or developing into an emotionally fraught search for a magic solution. Instead, the problem was identified, explained and discussed with Anna—unlike with Sophie (3.4), when we had no idea about how to understand the problem. As a result, Anna and I were able to move on to enjoy a 12-year marriage, despite the fact that there was no quick-fix—or even a long-term fix, for that matter.

xviii.   I believe that Anna and I were able move on with the marriage because we both had secure attachments that we could rely on. Anna, I believe, was securely attached within herself as the result of good parenting in her infancy, whereas I was in the process of *earning* security through my 'cultural revolution'—but more especially through my increasing commitment to sixth-form teaching, which was now becoming an institutional attachment, providing a secure base for me. This meant that we had enough personal and emotional resources to enjoy an affectionate relationship, even though it was no longer a sexual relationship. But there was another factor too.

xix.   This further factor was that, right from the outset, we committed ourselves to engage in joint projects—in which we sublimated our unspent sexual energy (7.8-9). The first of these was getting Anna settled into UK life, with meaningful work and British citizenship. Alongside that was our international travel project, with at least two European holidays or short breaks per year. Within three years came our decision to renovate and upgrade our home and after that, project USA—with trips to Florida, New York and then coast-to-coast. These projects were ongoing and free-flowing, one after the other. We didn't think for a second about what might happen to our relationship, if and when these creative projects suddenly dried up, or when, for example, I eventually retired. But as events transpired, they did dry up and we were soon forced to start some serious rethinking.

*

To support positive mental health:

1.   Going online to meet new people is a risky business. We all know this but it's an irresistible aspect of our present culture that we do so. We can't turn the clock back to pre-Internet days. Of course, the vast majority of online communications are beneficial to individuals and society in millions of different ways. But personal one-to-one communication with strangers carries particular risks. In my case, I was scammed for cash by one lady and touted for (illegal) 'marriages of

convenience' by two others. I was lucky—others have fared far worse—and people's mental health has been ruined as a result.

2. For optimum mental health in this respect, physical and real (not virtual) relationships are by far the best. So treasure and develop those you have and don't let the virtual world get in their way.

3. Furthermore, by understanding the nature of one's own attachment status, we can be more self-aware and self-accepting of our particular difficulties without the need to beat ourselves up about it or fall into deep and unnecessary misunderstandings with our partner.

Chapter 8 ~ Retirement Crises
2011–2018

1. Family Requiem
March 2011

"The day thou gavest, Lord, is ended,
The darkness falls at Thy behest"

Order of Service for Mum's funeral

My brother Nigel and I are both staying at Mum's otherwise empty bungalow in Coventry to decide on an Order of Service for her funeral, among other things. Mum had passed away shortly after her 95th birthday, having suffered a series of falls that had landed her in hospital, where she caught pneumonia, from which she did not recover.

There will be no Humanist service for Mum as we had arranged for Dad (6.5), for Mum had always been a believer, in a very Anglican sort of way. The funeral will be at *The Heart of England Crematorium*, near Nuneaton, the same place as for Dad. We choose two hymns: *The Lord's My Shepherd*, to open with, and *The Day Thou Gavest* at the end. As with Dad, I write the tribute and Nigel reviews it and adds some of his own memories. This time, I get the tone right straight away—it's not difficult as neither of us feel the same warmth towards Mum as we did towards Dad. The tricky bit is to avoid being hypocritical so we include a reference to her interference and fussing—always well intended—as well as to her goodness, kindness and courage, especially in the ten lonely years since Dad died. I also mention the 'Unforgettable Night' (1.1) that Mum told me about so often, and which seems to have clouded her life—and mine—ever since. I believe that her 'interference and fussiness' was, in fact, her attempt to make up for her unavailability as a young mother during the years she was clinically depressed.

There's no question that Mum was a good person at heart, even if she expressed this in ways that could seem to be overbearing. But in the tribute, we also reflect upon her unstinting work as our taxi-driver in our teenage years and the little appreciation we had shown at the time. Our parents must have been dismayed at how we had turned out: especially with me, becoming intensely religious and an Anglican minister, only to give it all up over a decade later. They would have been aghast at the thought that their child-rearing might have had something to do with this, although Mum had correctly identified, on more than one occasion, the problem that existed between us: "You and me, Jamie, we never seem to get on, do we? We're always at cross-purposes."

And precisely because of these difficulties, I felt at the time that no good purpose would be served by my trying to explain to her about maternal deprivation and insecure attachment. It would just fill her with even more self-pity than she already had, and make a difficult relationship even worse.

*

We believe that the funeral service hits the right note for the many relatives and friends present, and all goes according to plan. Again, I wanted to read the tribute myself, but the fear of breaking down caused me to be hyper-anxious, so I left it to the officiating minister. Nigel and I arrange for a plaque to mark the place in the crematorium grounds where our parents' ashes are scattered, which I intend to visit when I'm down that way, to pay my respects and leave new flowers.

After the funeral, there's a great deal to sort out concerning our parents' estate. It's the end of a Family, not just the end of Mum. Nigel does sterling work in sorting out the complex finances and putting the bungalow up for sale—it's an arduous task and he gives me regular printed updates of his progress. As for me, I head for Mum's large box of ill-assorted photos—over a thousand—and decide to make a family history out of them: "100 Years. The Milner-Adams Family: 1911-2011". In the end, I produce four, large, square volumes in black, embossed in gold. Even Nigel is impressed and says so: "It's a remarkable job you've done there—something to be proud of." It's the first compliment that I ever remember receiving from him—and it will probably be the last. So it's noted and treasured!

School is sympathetic as always and I'm given leave of absence for two weeks without question.

I cope much better with Mum's passing than with Dad's, as I always thought I would, especially now with Anna's support. We receive many cards of condolence, including one from my Year 13 sociology class, which is signed by every one of the fourteen students—it's very touching.

At this point, I had no idea that, by the end of the year, they would be signing another card—this time for me—on the occasion of *my* sudden passing—from school and into retirement—another Requiem of sorts.

2. A Fond Farewell
December 2011–June 2012

GOOD LUCK, JAMIE BOY!
WE LOVE YOU!
FROM YOUR AMAZIN' PHILOSOPHY GROUP!

*

After returning from my Amtrak coast-to-coast holiday in the USA (7.9), I make a huge decision: my next school year will be my last! I've already worked for eighteen months beyond the normal retirement age for teachers, mainly due to my timetable of only sixth-form work: 'A' level sociology, psychology and the philosophy of religion—with not a single disruptive lower-school class in sight! I love the work I'm doing! I love the intellectual challenge and my interactions with the bright, sparky students, who keep me on my toes—as well as sharing in their fun and good humour. All this makes me feel alive and keeps me young. Okay, young-ish.

However, in my school, as in most schools, there is an opposite force at work: *stress*. It comes in many guises, the most obvious being the demand from senior staff for continual, year-on-year improvement in results, especially at 'A' level. To achieve this, students have to be micro-managed: if Sarah only achieves a 'B' instead of an 'A' for an internal exam, there will be a thorough investigation of this particular 'failure' and an individual progress plan put in place to ensure there is no repeat. The focus is almost entirely on the teaching staff being responsible for student achievement. The fact that Sarah has been ill, or has suffered a family bereavement, or has skimped on her revision are not acceptable reasons for her 'under-achievement'. The question is always: what is the *teacher* going to do about it? With almost a hundred students and three other staff in my department, the workload and expectations are immense and unrealistic and, in some instances, clearly unfair. But things are about to get worse.

316

After the October half-term, new, more stringent lesson observations will be introduced and I soon see the effect of this on other teaching staff. Early one morning, I notice Mrs James—a superb psychology teacher—in tears, because she had failed to ask a question to each and every one of her twenty students during a lesson observation. She had missed one out! This resulted in her otherwise 'outstanding' lesson being classified as only 'good'. She thinks this is very unfair and so do I. We protest, but to no avail. This incident triggers my decision to bring forward my retirement to Christmas.

A few days later, I have a similar experience, which confirms my decision. With me, the 'problem' is my teaching style, which is discursive and creative and has served the students well for over two decades. The current demand is that all teaching should be formulaic and highly structured—jumping through hoops—and the hoops keep on multiplying! My Year 12 sociology lesson is judged 'unsatisfactory' because I missed out some hoops altogether! Again, I protest, and receive a sympathetic hearing from the Head. I inform her of my decision to retire at Christmas, and my repeat lesson observation is deferred until after my retirement date—so it will never happen. It's a fair compromise—for I've no wish to leave a successful teaching career under a cloud, being another victim of the current trend for over-regulation.

*

During my final week, various students come to wish me well in retirement, and some express sadness at my sudden and impending departure. Several give me cards and other gifts and we have some informal class photos taken. There's a similar reaction from the staff, many of whom are caught in the same dilemma as me, but without having retirement as their way out.

Eventually, my final lesson arrives—it's a senior philosophy of religion class. The students have planned a retirement party for me: they will bring some food and Christmas crackers, and I will bring the music and drinks. We enjoy some pop videos and sing along to Britney Spears' *Till the World Ends*—as mine is about to, within the next thirty minutes! Suddenly, Mrs James pops in from next door and takes me into the corridor to chat. When I return, the students shout 'Happy Retirement!' and direct my gaze to a hastily hung banner on the wall. It reads:

GOOD LUCK, JAMIE BOY! WE LOVE YOU! FROM YOUR AMAZIN' PHILOSOPHY GROUP!

I am deeply touched, especially as I'm really leaving them in the lurch, with their final 'A' level exams only six months away. Indeed, a couple of them mention the 'abandonment issues' that I'm causing them but they seem to bear me no ill-will—in fact, quite the opposite. Miranda presents me with chocolates and wine from the group, together with a couple of cards, one of them rather large. All too soon, the final bell sounds and there are hugs all around as they troop out, some with a cheery 'Happy Christmas', others with 'I'll miss you'. I shall certainly miss them.

For a few minutes, I stand in the classroom alone—for the final time. I think of the hundreds of lively discussions and serious questions, the banter and good humour that have made this ordinary-looking classroom such a treasured place to be. I see the colourful posters of Marx, Durkheim, Descartes and Freud, to be discussed no more—at least by me. I leave the room, shut the door, return to the staffroom, then home to Anna, with my thoughts and my loss.

*

At home, I relax in an armchair, surrounded by cards and Christmas decorations; the cards are not Christmas cards, but retirement cards, mainly from students, and they are mounting in number. I open the envelopes given to me during my last lesson—and I'm taken aback by what I find. The large card contains almost 60 student signatures. But they are not just signatures—as almost all have included personal expressions about myself and my teaching. They are overwhelmingly affirmative and affectionate. They thank me for my lessons, which have been *'interesting'*, *'knowledgeable'*, *'wise'* and *'fun'*! Again and again, I'm thanked for being an *'amazing'* teacher who will be sorely missed:

"You've been an amazing teacher, one of the best, most knowledgeable teachers I've had. I'm going to miss you loads. Love from Amy. xxx" is typical of many.

As is Bradley's: *"There's no way I could have passed AS philosophy if it wasn't for you. Thank you for your wisdom—from Plato to Made in Chelsea! You're a great teacher! Brad. xx"*

I can scarcely believe what I'm reading! I had often received 'thank you' cards from various individuals and 'A' level groups and I had always thought that I had a fairly good rapport with most of my classes—but not to this extent. And I certainly had *never* thought of myself as an *amazing* teacher with such a clear personal impact on so many. Now that it's all over, I'm struggling to hold back the tears at what I'm reading—and at the good, warm wishes expressed by so many towards me. I never knew that I was appreciated or valued so much—until now.

*

In the New Year, I spend the first few weeks in a daze. Anna is out at work all day, and I do very little, other than buy a daily paper and then go to a local fitness centre for some swimming and gym-work. I'm totally bored and I'm constantly wondering how things are going at school and how my replacement teacher is coping. She should be okay as she is well qualified, and I had given her substantial materials and support after she had accepted the job.

Then, in mid-March and completely out of the blue, I receive a phone call from my former line-manager.

"Jamie, unfortunately your replacement teacher has left. She couldn't handle the job. Is there any chance you could come out of retirement for a few months and help prepare the senior classes for their final 'A' level exams in June?"

I'm stunned, but highly delighted to be asked back and be given the chance to thank the students for their kind words and cards. But only on one condition! That I'm allowed to teach the way I want to teach, which is clearly appreciated by the students, judging from the comments in their cards. In other words, I'll not be subject to any Ofsted-style, hoop-jumping lesson observations. Or indeed, any observations at all. If I'm given that assurance, I will come back immediately. An hour later, my line manager calls back to say that my request has been unanimously agreed by senior staff—they just want me back, to give the students the best chance they have of getting good results.

I am welcomed back by my classes like a conquering hero! It's a chance to make it up to those who felt that I had abandoned them, which I had felt guilty about. Several staff congratulate me for refusing to subject myself to the bureaucratic diktats of Ofsted-like observations, which, in our view, undermine the professional judgements of teachers and their control over their own lessons.

In class, I immediately get on with the task in hand—improving those topics where my replacement teacher had fallen short and consolidating the whole of the year's work through thorough revision. By the time the exams arrive, the majority of students have regained their confidence and, overall, their eventual results are in line with their predicted grades—some a bit better, others a bit worse—as is usually the case.

*

Before the summer term ends, I am invited—almost press-ganged—by the senior students into attending their 'Leavers' Ball' at a local hotel. The boys are there in their smart suits and the girls in their posh frocks. Inevitably, I am urged to take to the dance floor despite the fact that my solo dad-dancing is not up to my modern jive style! I'm acutely aware, however, that this time, it is the end— the very end—of my sixth-form teaching career and I don't want to look into the abyss…

I'm reluctant to give up so much friendship, acceptance and warmth, so I stay right to the end of the evening and give out my contact details to any student who might want to use me as a future reference. At midnight, we're all thrown out, with a few students being the worse for drink. Once outside, some boys come over to shake my hand and several girls come over for a final hug. It's been an excellent evening and very emotional all round—both for the students as well as for myself.

It's the end of school life for them and their years of companionship—and the end of a thirty-four-year teaching career for me.

And so, for all of us, things are about to change.

3. Things have Changed
Bob Dylan [129]
2012–3

After the high of the Leavers' Ball, I'm not surprised to find myself crashing down to a new low now that I've no more sixth-form classes to teach—ever. Fortunately, a flurry of text messages restores my equilibrium: two students get in touch. Miranda: to arrange to meet for a coffee and a chat about her results and Jake invites me to his campus at Leicester University in the new term once he has settled in. I feel a bit better—the bonds have not been completely broken.

Then, a few days later, I hear from Nigel that Mum's bungalow has been sold at last so that the estate can now be divided equally between us. I inform Anna about this and we both agree to put my house on the market and use the new funds to buy something larger, more rural and nearer to Nottingham, where Anna has been working at the university for the past year. She can do with a shorter commute!

This provides us with our next exciting project—searching for a new home in a new location—and we talk of little else! Events move very quickly, and we soon have interested buyers for our house. Each weekend and some evenings, we tour the Nottingham area for our new home and soon spot a house in the commuter village of Ruddington, south of Nottingham, with Rushcliffe Country Park on our doorstep. It's a modern, three-bedroom detached house, with a mature English garden and a beautiful lawn. It's the garden that sells itself to us. On a bright summer's day, the garden has that 'Wow!' factor and we're both hooked! Typical of my 'free-child' spirit, I make an immediate offer, before anyone else views it. The offer is accepted and, given a fair wind, we should be able to move in during my October half-term. Except I don't have an October half-term any more. I forgot.

The purchase price allows us a bit of wiggle room with our finances as the house needs some improvements. We make plans to convert the third bedroom into a larger bathroom, with the current small bathroom becoming a meditation room for Anna. We will also convert the attached garage into an office, with a downstairs toilet and extra storage space. Finally, we will add a conservatory with under-floor heating, where we can relax in both summer and winter.

Fortunately, we know a guy at our dance class who specialises in this sort of work at a reasonable cost. So it's full steam ahead for a late October move, then at least four months of upheaval during the alterations. Exciting times! My parents would be well pleased with how we are using their estate. They would love the garden and house, apart from the stairs, of course. I feel that I'm reliving my father's post-war dream—a quiet life in a semi-rural location and with a beautiful garden to tend. It's a good feeling.

There's only one problem—with the house-purchase and alterations combined, we will completely empty our coffers! Anna offers to lend a few thousand pounds from her pension fund in order to get the job done so long as it's repaid. But it means no more trips to America, or anywhere else for that matter, for a very long time, as we tighten our belts. Instead, we will have a fabulous house to enjoy—come rain or shine!

Fortunately, I have enough money saved up in a separate account to take Ed to America the following Easter, for a musical treat to celebrate his band's latest CD production and to mark his 30th birthday.

*

Having fallen in love with Amtrak on my pre-retirement coast-to-coast trip across America, I am keen on another US rail trip—if Ed is agreeable. He certainly is when I tell him of Amtrak's *Jazz, Blues and Rock 'n' Roll* tour, which will take us to the music cities of Chicago, Memphis and New Orleans. Ed is well impressed and asks if we can add in a visit to New York with which to end the trip. Could we do that? Yes, we can!

Upon arriving in the Windy City after a direct flight from Manchester, we head for the shore of Lake Michigan and discover how windy it actually is, as a bitter blast cuts through us like a knife, forcing us to walk backwards to the city's Art Institute! For two evenings, we enjoy electric blues music at Buddy Guy's *Legends* club just behind our hotel. The following day, after a scary walk on the Sky-deck ledge up on Willis Tower, we're off to Union station to board *The City of New Orleans* for an evening meal and a top-deck sleeper cabin to Memphis, Tennessee. As we wait to board, I'm as excited as a little child!

*

Ten hours later we arrive in Memphis in pitch darkness and are whisked by shuttle-bus to our hotel for an early morning breakfast. We have two days to take in the sights and sounds of Beale Street, Sun Studios, Graceland, various music museums and the Lorraine Motel—the memorial to the assassination of Martin Luther King. Oh, and the marching ducks at the Peabody Hotel! Top of the pops, however, is undoubtedly Sun Studios, the birthplace of rock 'n' roll—where we stand on the same spot where Elvis first recorded, and Ed becomes Jerry Lee Lewis at the same piano where he first boogie-woogied *A Whole Lotta Shakin' Goin On'* and *Great Balls of Fire*!

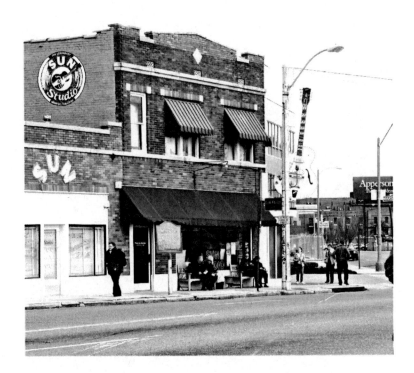

Sun Studios, Memphis—the birthplace of rock 'n roll

*

Amazingly, just forty-eight hours after our arrival, we're back on board *The City of New Orleans* for an early morning trip to *The Big Easy*, which is still in recovery eight years after the devastation of hurricane Katrina in 2005. As the train winds its way south through the Mississippi Delta, we feel the warmth of the surrounding swamplands and sight the occasional lazy alligator.

Soon, the skyscrapers of New Orleans appear on the horizon and before we know it, we're out under the city's blue skies, its balmy sunshine and gently waving palms. There's jazz playing on every street corner of the popular French Quarter and our taxi-driver warns us about the decadence of the infamous Bourbon Street—so that's exactly where we head off to, for our first night's entertainment! Godfather and godson, decadent together!

For the next four evenings, we attend various jazz or blues gigs, including a jive-dance to a jazz band for our final night, where I'm in my element! During the day, we take a trip along the Mississippi on a paddle-steamer and visit Congo Square—where Sunday afternoon slave-gatherings had drummed, danced and sang, and which had led to the city's current musical traditions. All too soon, it's back to the station to catch *The Crescent*—the overnight sleeper to New York— a mere thirty-hour journey away!

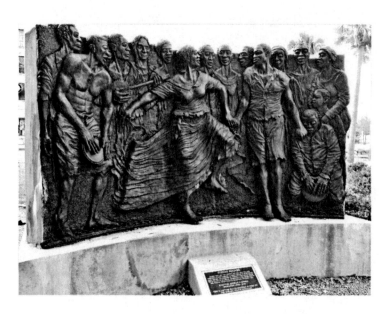

Congo Square, New Orleans—
the birthplace of Mardi Gras, jazz and rhythm& blues

*

Our Manhattan hotel is right next to the Empire State Building, so we're up to the top before we've even unpacked! In the next three days, we visit Times Square and then Central Park, wherein lies a memorial to John Lennon. We listen to Mahler's Third Symphony in Carnegie Hall, pay our respects to the victims of 9/11 at the impressive National Memorial and walk in the footsteps of Bob Dylan in Greenwich Village—including a fun mock-up of the cover of his *Freewheelin* album at the same Jones' Street location. I'm Bob Dylan (of course) and Ed, with his long hair and shorter stature, makes a passing resemblance to Suze Rotolo, Dylan's girlfriend at the time. It's a fitting symbol of our wonderful, freewheelin' trip!

Back home, we had already booked to see Bob Dylan himself in Blackpool, on his *Never Ending Tour* (7.9). So within a fortnight of our return, we're on our feet again for his encore of *All Along The Watchtower* and *Blowin' in the Wind*. After a few days spent with Ed, I return to our new Nottingham home and, with Anna out at work all day, there's only one thought that's blowing in the wind for me: *things have changed—big-time*.

*

There's lots to do around the house now that the workmen have left, and there's always Rushcliffe Country Park to explore, but there are no sixth-form classes for me to teach, no friendly faces to greet me each day and no new ideas for me to research. Suddenly I'm lost—completely lost.

I have plenty of time to think about my new situation—hours, days, weeks and months of nothingness, with ten or twenty years ahead—maybe more. My thoughts tell me that:

- I've no *motivation* for anything, except to eat to stay alive and relieve the boredom.
- I've no *enthusiasm* for anything, with the house now finished and Ed's holiday completed.
- I've no *intellectual challenge*, without students to challenge me.
- I've no *everyday social discourse*, except with Anna for a few minutes each day.
- I've no *familiar environment* and no known landmarks. It's all new.
- I've no *time-structure*—just a totally unstructured retirement wilderness.

All I have is Anna, an empty house and dance—it's not enough. Not nearly enough.

So I reformulate Bob Dylan's words for myself:

A lonely man with a hungry mind,
All his good times now left behind

Time hangs heavy now—for things have changed
[130].

4. The Search I
2013–5

I...have known the evenings, mornings, afternoons,
I have measured out my life with coffee spoons.
T. S. Eliot. *The Love Song of J. Alfred Prufrock* [131]

While my external world is delightful—a new house and garden with a Country Park next door—my inner world is bleak. In an attempt to cheer myself up, I set off for *Waterstones* in Nottingham to buy a book fitting for dedication to my parents, for their role in providing me with a good education. An education that had been the foundation of a successful and engaging career—even if it had been via a most circuitous of routes. It's my posthumous 'thank you' to them.

I choose an expensive hardback about the poems of T. S. Eliot, the wellspring of my reflective life and academic journeys [132]. After the purchase, I browse through it in the third-floor café, but I don't get past the second coffee before I give up. I *feel* like the isolated *Prufrock*, or an alienated character from *The Waste Land*, but I don't want to admit this—or the abyss into which I am falling. It's similar with my other books, especially those I used for teaching—they've lost their power to thrill. They're like engines without fuel so I take them to a charity shop where they may find a more useful life. There's no looking backwards—I need to move forwards if I can.

*

Through the rest of the summer, while Anna's out at work, I take myself off to Rushcliffe Country Park. I'm happy to be using my new bike, bought from mother's estate. Perhaps I should join a cycling club? I'll look into it. I enjoy the novelty of exploring new places—for the first few trips at least. I notice the variety of trees in the park—they're beautiful and interesting and perhaps have potential. I'll become a tree-hugger! Or just an everyday naturalist. Perhaps. I could be a volunteer gardener at the Park—there's so many things I could do! But I suddenly remember that our own garden needs weeding, which I promised Anna I'd see to.

Over tea in the conservatory, I notice the birds on an old feeder: blue tits, great tits, a robin—and that beautiful liquid song of goldfinches! I know a bit about birds, because Nigel's a birdwatcher and I've learnt a bit from him. I'll become a twitcher! Or just an ordinary bird-watcher—so I start making a list of all our garden birds. Then there's the Park birds too. I buy a small recorder and record some birdsong in the field. Nigel will tell me who's singing what, and that he does. Anna finds a young goldfinch on the ground, who's flown into our kitchen window, so I look after for him for a week in the conservatory—until he's fit to fly again. I enjoy that—something meaningful for me to do at last!

Then Anna comes up with a great idea! A bird of our own—especially one we can train! We buy a young cockatiel, bright yellow—he's beautiful! But there's an unforeseen problem. We have a cage, but I have a conscience: birds are not for caging! So I allow him to fly free in the house and before long, every surface is covered with newspaper to catch his mess—dust, feathers and poo! It's a disastrous experiment and after six months, we return one very untrained bird to the pet shop from whence he came.

I start to realise that I'm missing *people*. Birds, trees and gardens are all very well, but they don't really do it for me. I learn about Nottingham's *Sunday Assembly*—a non-religious Sunday morning gathering—and I'm an immediate convert, even joining the organising committee for a while. But these committee guys are young and hi-tech, and I don't seem to fit the profile. And every Sunday gathering is a one-off. It lacks continuity and any intrinsic community so I'm lonely in a crowd and soon drop out. Perhaps it also reminds me of the bad old days of church.

Friends tell me that I should join U3A—the University of the Third Age— and so I do. Table-tennis on a Monday morning seems a good start to the week— but it doesn't last. I don't want to identify myself with such elderly folk who, although well-skilled, just play for fun each week, without any league table or competitive edge. So it's back to the house and garden—and in the afternoons…I measure out my life with coffee spoons.

5. The Search II
2013–5

Once you wake up and smell the coffee,
it's hard to go back to sleep [133]

I can do with some extra cash but my state pension is not available for another couple of years. Therefore, during the summer, I send off letters to five local schools, asking them if they need any exam invigilators. I also offer lessons in Transactional Analysis if any are interested. As it happens, my nearest school is interested in both: an invigilator for forthcoming January exams, and some T.A. for the Year 11 students. This feels like progress.

I undertake the basic training for an invigilator's role, along with half a dozen others. And I'm invited to deliver the TA lessons in the spring term and on a voluntary basis. I wonder what I've let myself in for with these unknown students—but I needn't worry. The lessons work their old magic and I have no discipline problems; I receive a number of appreciative comments. My only pay is for the exam work but perhaps the TA lessons have earned me some brownie points. As for the invigilation—I think I'll die of boredom! And there are no coffee breaks!

Later on, I receive an email, informing me of a sixth-form supervisor's post at the school. It's part-time, non-teaching, casual employment and poorly paid— but I'm definitely interested!

I apply, am interviewed and appointed to one of the two posts available, to start the following academic year. It's a godsend! I'm back in a familiar sixth-form environment and although my job is to ensure the students' silent study, there's chance for some football banter between lessons or with those students that I'm not supervising. It's good that my weeks have some structure at last, but my inner core of emptiness remains as I continue to live a life without meaning.

*

The week before Christmas, I learn that Curly's wife, Joanna—a lovely lady and a long-standing confidante—has passed away after her fight with cancer. Naturally, I'm very upset and attend her funeral, at which I meet up with some old school pals. In the New Year, Curly, in need of some company and support, invites me for a weekend at his St Alban's home. His hospitality is generous as always—then, after coffee: "Do you fancy a game of Subbuteo? I've still got all the stuff!"

My face lights up! I'd played this game of table football throughout my teenage years, right up till my evangelical conversion, when I became overly serious and gave it up as child's play. But now, the green open spaces of the Subbuteo cloth and the flicks, kicks and goal-keeping saves of the plastic players immediately appeal! Curly and I had been equally matched competitors in virtually every sport—and clearly nothing has changed in the intervening years. We play a 5-game series, taking turns to be Coventry City—and I'm immediately re-converted! I will buy a new set of everything and use our new conservatory as my stadium to play in. I'm in passionate 'free child' mode once more—and this is the first chink of light in my ongoing retirement crisis.

Back home in Nottingham, I devise my own Subbuteo league and work out how I can play against myself. I also discover a local Subbuteo club where I'm given good advice about purchasing the best quality components for my new fun enterprise. However, after attending the club for a few weeks, I find the guys there are far too serious, hyper-critical and enslaved by myriads of rules and regulations. It's absolutely no *fun* at all—and it's definitely not for me! But the game itself definitely is!

*

I continue to dance, but without any great enthusiasm. I'm still lost and empty inside, still missing my sixth-form students and the dynamics of teaching. If anything, I'd prefer to talk than dance to make up for the near-continuous conversations of sixth-form lessons. Anna and I don't talk as much, now that we don't have a common project on the go, and on Friday nights, I attend dances alone as she's too tired after a hard, working week.

One Friday night in September, I dance for the first time with Jessie, who's very chatty. She's young-looking, slim and pretty, with natural long blonde hair. She's a good dancer too! By the end of the evening, we've danced and talked quite a lot. She's very open, and it's become apparent that we're both in marriages that seem unsatisfactory for a variety of different reasons. For me, there's an attraction to Jessie that I can't quite identify—but I soon realise what it is when I recognise her cheery greeting at the next dance.

"Hi Jamie, so what are we doing today then? A bit of blues?"

"We're dancing hard, with a smile!" is my instant reply. Now where did that come from? (7.9) I suddenly realise why I'm drawn to Jessie—she's like my bright and bubbly sixth-form students! And from that moment on, I don't miss my students so much because Jessie symbolically represents them. Thereafter, through emails, texts and dances—and our discussions on psychology and football (she's a Nottingham Forest fan)—I start to become emotionally attached to Jessie. Nevertheless, I remain bleak and empty in my core and nothing touches that—although my friendship with Jessie is giving me a buzz—just as my sixth-form classes used to do—though for different reasons.

With autumn gathering pace and evenings drawing in, I begin to wonder whether Anna and I will arrange anything special to mark my approaching 65th birthday—and my ignominious entry into official old age. I think it should be marked, and indeed it is—but not in the way I expect. For in the middle of November, Anna announces her plans to attend a meditation ashram in India the following month—if that's alright by me. Her meditation is important to her and her hard work deserves a holiday so, of course, I agree. But it means she'll be away for my birthday, which is disappointing—although she'll leave a card and present all wrapped up before she flies off.

After taking her to Stansted, on the journey home, my bleakness increases about my forthcoming birthday with its prospect of a meal-for-one and coffee in front of the TV. I email Jessie: "How do you fancy going to a Christmas dinner-dance for my birthday?"

"Thanks! Yes, I do—let's see if I can wangle it! And I'll get back to you!"

So Jessie 'wangles' another dance-night away from her husband—he's getting used to it by now.

We arrive at our table for two inside a sparkling and festive ballroom—shared with other Christmas revellers, some danceable music and an uplifting party mood! Doubtless Anna is enjoying her ashram—and I'm enjoying my unexpected birthday treat! Jessie and I leave the party at midnight, with a smile, a hug and a kiss on the cheek—she's saved my day!

As my 65th birthday had approached, I learnt that I was due to receive a church pension for my three years in a Lincolnshire parish (2.6) almost 40 years previously. It would consist of a small monthly pension—and a large lump sum! I'm amazed! All useful funds—for we still need to renew some windows and I can now completely refurbish my bedroom—the only room so far untouched.

I decide to transform my bedroom into *Café Pop*—where I can entertain friends with coffee, food and music. I set it up like a café with facilities such as a kettle and small table, cushions for my bed-settee, with a brand new music centre and a turntable for my vinyl records, both old and new. Stone-effect wallpaper will display miniature guitars and pop memorabilia—such as Abba's autographs, famous LP sleeves, programmes from Britney and Katy Perry concerts and a large poster of Bob Dylan from his Blackpool gig. I can add more later. I find it both amusing and fitting that 50 years after I'd given my entire pop collection to charity—as 'the music of the devil' (2.3)—the church gives me a lump sum that enables me to get it all back again—and more besides! I still feel bleak and without purpose but I'm also feeling more uniquely myself—and not so much part of a couple.

*

After a decade without contact, I meet up with Kevin Milburn at a former colleague's retirement party. We've football and religion in common and I well remember his support for me in my early difficult days at school (5.1). But we've another connection: we were contemporaries at Durham and although I don't remember him, he remembers me. We agree to meet in Durham for coffee in the cathedral Refectory. But first, I've a pilgrimage to make—a sacred site to see.

I find the green-roofed Appleby lecture theatre where, 46 years previously, my naïve evangelical faith had been swept aside within the hour (2.4). The theatre looks much the same, so I try the external door and enter. I push the internal door and it swings open with all the lights flicking on! A cleaning lady says I can take my time, and I do. I sit on the same wooden bench, halfway back, and relive those ancient, dark moments. I reflect on the academic, intellectual and emotional journeys that Dr Sargant's lecture set in train. Theology, philosophy, sociology, psychology and Attachment—it all started here, in principle, for me. This is my pilgrimage—to this ordinary, yet extraordinary and historic place. Historic for me, that is—where, so painfully, I had been forced to grow up. Or at least make a start.

I had used to think that Durham had imprisoned my mind (4.5). But now, as I continue to sit and reflect, another, more positive image comes to mind—*a crucible*. I start to realise that, in the fiery white heat of my turbulent times at Durham, a melting pot had poured forth the key elements necessary for a long and successful career in teaching the social sciences. In particular, I recognise that this crucible had led me to develop:

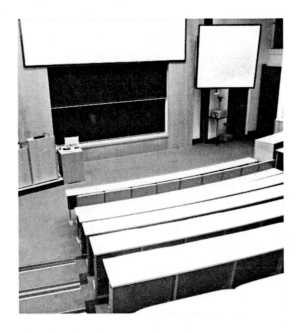

Back inside the Appleby lecture theatre,
46 years later, and with a new perspective.

   (a) A new methodology of evidence-based rational thought
   (b) New areas of interest in the social sciences and wider culture

And so, deep in thought, I leave the theatre in silence and head for the Cathedral Refectory where I push open the glass door, spot Kevin Milburn and smell the coffee.

6. The Black Hole

Easter 2016

"Jamie, when you're in a hole…"

The first phase of my post-retirement search for meaning was little more than measuring out my life in coffee spoons—there was simply no meaningful existence to be had (8.4). The second phase (8.5) felt slightly better as it provided me with symbolic renewals of key developmental milestones that connected me to a meaningful past—a past of football, pop, girls, university experience and a fulfilling teaching career.

However, throughout all these post-retirement years, I continue to feel lost, bleak and depressed—nothing, it seems, will shift. To be sure, a game of Subbuteo with Curly or some jive-dancing with Jessie will temporarily lift my spirits, but my underlying mood remains the same.

However, things are about to change—though not in a good way.

*

Anna and I decide that we need a break. Anna has been struggling with her new job, with its demanding deadlines and long hours, and I feel that a change of scenery might do me good as well—especially a spot of sunshine! So we book ourselves on a week's dance holiday on the Costa del Sol. I'm a little wary, as I'd been on two dance-holidays before: one had been great (6.8), but the other had not (7.4) so I hoped for the best.

After arriving at our sea-view hotel, the inaugural 'housekeeping' meeting for our 70-strong group is scheduled for 5 pm. But as I cast my eye around the room, I get a severe shock: *everyone is old*! And that includes me! The only exceptions are Anna and the bar-staff. I know many of the dancers there but I now see them as they really are, without the darkness of the dance hall or the masks of mascara airbrushing away a thousand wrinkles. I'm shocked for several reasons:

1. Because, de facto, I'm now part of the silver generation of senior citizens—and I'm being forced to acknowledge this fact, which I absolutely refuse to do! Peter Pan is still alive and kicking within!
2. At dances back home, there's normally a wide age-spectrum, from 30-year olds upwards—and I tend to dance with the younger end, but I'm now stuck with a load of 'oldies', which also includes me! It's a most unpleasant double-whammy, including my self-acknowledgement of my ageist prejudices.

On top of my pre-existing depression, this is too much to bear and I tell Anna so. I want to be on the next plane home but financially, that's not possible and in any case, Anna wants to stay. I therefore have to grit my teeth and carry on, as I start to slip into the abyss of clinical depression once more. My mood is lifted somewhat by Anna's support and by our day-trips to Gibraltar and Malaga. And by Jessie's daily texts. Otherwise, the trip is a nightmare. I'm in a hole again and in need of help!

*

Back home, things are no better—one can't just wish, or dance, such depression away. However, I delay a trip to the doctor's for two reasons. Firstly, I already have a supply of tablets from an earlier time that give me a temporary lift. Secondly, before the holiday, I met Nancy at a dance. She's a well-qualified psychotherapist, masseuse and fan of Attachment Theory! So I wonder if she can help.

Nancy is young, warm, charming and tactile. Her soothing massages help shut out the darkness for a while and we also talk about my search for meaning, my attachment history—and Jessie. She tells me what I already know—but it comes with a twist.

"Jamie, there's no quick fix, so I won't pretend there is. But I do suggest that you stop trying to get a quick fix for yourself."

"So what are you saying exactly?"

"I'm suggesting that you stop searching around for some activity or other that you hope is going to put things right: becoming a cyclist, a birdwatcher or other bird-brained ideas. You're only making things worse. Jamie, when you're in a hole, stop digging new ones."

Nancy also advises me to continue with my scrapbooks and chart-work, because they are creative and rewarding. But I should stop looking for a 'magic moment' that will resolve my post-retirement blues. I need to let go, enjoy the smaller pleasures of life and accept that a 'magic moment' is most unlikely to happen. In time, something may emerge. I accept what Nancy is saying but it doesn't exactly thrill me—and it feels very scary to 'let go' of trying to fix things.

I sense that she's absolutely right about this but, as things turn out, she's also very wrong!

7. A Magic Moment
Summer 2016

I continue to see Nancy, for both massage and therapy, every two weeks. It's my only high spot in the midst of my depression. She continues to encourage my creativity, especially after I bring along some of my work to one of our sessions.

Following our meeting in Durham, Kevin Milburn invites me to stay for a weekend with him and his wife in their house—a large town house—in Newcastle. We can do some more catching up and also go to a match as he's a Newcastle United season-ticket holder. It's a very kind offer that I soon take up. I travel by train to Newcastle where, in the middle of my first night, I wake to a recurring thought—perhaps triggered by his hospitality—namely that I DO have support from a number of sources, despite my feelings of isolation. I'm not on my own, as I often tend to think. Finding a pen and paper at 3 am, I start to construct TEAM JAMIE SUPPORT—a football team consisting of myself, my friends and other supportive associates…

As the only one with ultimate responsibility for my life, I have to be the goalkeeper. In front of me are the stout defenders of Curly, Katie, Angelique and Anna. For my midfielders, I have my new school; Kevin Milburn; Coventry City and Ed. Jessie and Nancy are my up-front strikers—yes, it's a 4-4-2 system! I also write some pen-pictures for us all, as if for a 1960s matchday programme—but very tongue-in-cheek. For example:

Curly: A robust and reliable defender, Curly is the longest serving member of the team. What he might now lack in pace and agility, he more than makes up for in experience. He clears the ball well and is always looking over his shoulder to help out the dodgy goalkeeper.

I enjoy the feelings of support and fun, and sleep follows quickly thereafter. I realise that it's only masking the depression but what I don't realise at the time, is that it's the next step of a therapeutic process.

On my return trip, at Newcastle station, I buy an interesting-sounding book: *Retirement: the Psychology of Reinvention* [134]. As a result, I start to see that my teaching career developed into a 'career attachment' and the result of that is my experience of retirement as a 'career bereavement'. No wonder I'm in crisis and still depressed almost five years after teaching my last lesson. This is all very interesting, but it does nothing to shift my low mood on the journey home.

Sitting opposite me on the train is a Japanese student who is engrossed in a paperback, the covers of which are all white with an orange sticker on the front. I'm intrigued so I enquire about her book. "Oh yes, it's great—you should read it sometime. It's called *Quiet*." [135]

*

The following weekend, I buy a copy and once started, I can't put it down! It's about the Introversion-Extroversion spectrum, something that had never appeared on the AQA psychology syllabus at school. I had briefly come across it in the philosophy of religion course, in connection with Carl Jung—but it was not directly relevant. In any case, I couldn't personally make any sense of it. Am I an Extravert—being 'God's evangelist' and an up-front teacher? Or am I an Introvert—loving the solitude of reading and being pretty hopeless in certain social situations?

After completing the 20-question test set by author Susan Cain, I am left in no doubt. I score 14/20 towards the Introversion end of the spectrum, and the rest of the book supports this result. So I'm an Introvert who has good acting skills for when I need them—for preaching and teaching, and for enthusing about such passions as Coventry City or modern jive dancing.

I'm so engrossed that I read it cover-to-cover over the weekend, then arrive, fired up by my new discovery, at a local U3A psychology meeting [136] on Monday morning. The group's leader has chosen a TED talk for the morning's discussion and to my complete astonishment, it's Susan Cain again, a self-declared Introvert, talking to a thousand people about the virtues of being an Introvert in an Extroverted (American) society! It's a complete coincidence and

I can hardly believe my luck! Is somebody trying to tell me something? It's probably my unconscious again, trying to get through to me.

I think the group is rather impressed with my fresh and detailed knowledge of Susan Cain's book! And there's another thing: the Introversion-Extroversion continuum seems to have nothing to do with Attachment! Now *that's* a thought that knocks me sideways and rocks my mental world—but I'm still depressed. It's hanging over me like a winter's fog.

*

Ten days later, I'm watching a BBC4 programme in the *Great Minds* series, presented by Bettany Hughes. The programmes on Marx and Nietzsche have been excellent. Now it's Freud's turn. During the programme, there is, inevitably, reference to the Freud-Jung friendship, their diverging approaches and their acrimonious split. It's about halfway through the hour-long programme when two words suddenly flash into my mind like a lightning bolt:

Creative Psychology!

That's it! I exclaim to myself. *That's it! That's what I'll do! It's brilliant!*

It's a Magic Moment! An 'Aha' experience! A Damascus-road conversion! Yes, another one.

*

I rush upstairs to tell Anna. She's pleased for me but doesn't really know what to make of it—until I tell her something else: "My depression—it's completely gone! I feel absolutely fine! And I know what I'm going to do with the rest of my life!"

"What's that?"

"I'm going to do Creative Psychology!"

"So what does that mean?"

I try to explain—I've already worked it out:

"Creative Psychology is a continuum. At one end, there's pure creativity—like the family photo albums I made after Mum died. At the other end, there's pure academic psychology, like some of the big textbooks on Attachment Theory that I buy. But in between, there's a combination of both. My creativity can be psychological—combining pictures and charts with psychological analysis, for example. And my psychology can be creative and open-ended. I've now come to realise that there's a lot of psychology that's NOT about Attachment."

The following morning, I'm up early to trace the wellsprings of Creative Psychology: the creativity aspect I can trace back to my scrapbooks and to my Chart Therapy after the *McVicar* programme in 1989 (4.5). The psychology aspect I can trace back to the *Battle for the Mind* lecture in 1969, which seemed so destructive at the time (2.4). Both aspects have their sources in Durham: it was a crucible—rather than a prison—after all.

As for the more recent triggers: it's Nancy who encouraged my creativity and suggested that my creative reflections went back to my teenage years and to T. S. Eliot. Even then, she suggests, I was more, and deeper, than just football, pop and girls. And it's Susan Cain who opened my mind to a new psychology that goes well beyond the bounds of both exam board specifications and Attachment Theory. I symbolise these converging streams on an A4-size chart, showing the various connections through time, with photographs of the main places and players involved.

Creative psychology has lift off!

*

The next eighteen months see me involved in an outpouring of new analysis, new charts, new reflections and new photos, with titles such as:

- *Retirement as career bereavement: readings from psychology*
- *Post-retirement blues: 2011-6*
- *Life's unfolding ladder: 1950-2017*
- *Top 10 'Aha!' and 'Oh no!' moments: 1950-2017*
- *40 positive lessons from romantic rejections—and rejectings*

By the time I've 'finished' in late 2017, I've an 80-page presentation file, full of material, labelled simply: *Creative Psychology: 2016-7*. Of course, it will never be finished, for Creative Psychology is an ongoing and unending series of projects, both big and small—so long as I have a brain to think, eyes to see and a computer to cut and paste.

*

However, at the same time that Creative psychology (and a renewed retirement) is taking off, a former project—the Russian revolution—is in the process of shutting down. My new love for Creative psychology is departing the station for destinations unknown—as for my marriage to Anna, it's coming to the end of the line.

8. The End of the Line
2016–7

"Jamie, I want a divorce! There are three people in our marriage and it's rather crowded. You're more attached to Jessie than to me!"

I try to deny Anna's accusations, but I don't sound very convincing—I know she's probably right. My friendship with Jessie has never been physical—never anything more than a peck on the cheek. But there are emotional attachments, though stronger on my side than hers.

Our marital problems go a long way back and run deep. But Anna isn't interested in that. She's only interested in what she sees as the problem now—and that's *Jessie!* As far as Anna is concerned—herself a huge admirer of Princess Diana—Jessie is the evil Camilla and I'm the unfaithful Charles, while Anna can hold her head up high as the loyal, devoted and loving Diana—the wronged and deeply hurt victim. And that's all there is to it. It makes perfect sense. Simples!

*

I can understand why Anna sees things this way, but it doesn't mean it's the *only* way of seeing things. Anna is not wrong about what she feels and sees etched in my face—but my issue is that she sees too little rather than too much. Anna is only interested in a powerful, highly focussed picture of our marriage, whereas I'm more interested in the widescreen view, the broader picture, that has given rise to this particular situation. I believe that this larger picture contains four main features, which have contributed to a marriage that, in Anna's eyes, has become 'rather crowded':

1. From the start of our honeymoon in the UK, the dramatic change in our sexual relationship posed a problem and was always likely to present a

threat (7.7). At one point, after three years of marriage, we did think about splitting up, though remain partners—but in the end, neither of us wanted that (7.8). But it does show that our problems go a long way back.

2. The reason, I believe, why our marriage has been outwardly 'successful' was that we have both sublimated our sexual energy into meaningful joint projects that have enriched both of our lives (7.8-9). We had 'Beaten the Blues'—or so it seemed. However, upon the purchase of, and with alterations to, our new house in south Nottingham (8.3), we ran out of money and joint projects at the time when we needed them most: my retirement. This meant that without a new project binding us together, our new external circumstances were more likely to drive us apart.

3. It was not long after our resettlement in south Nottingham that Anna gained a new and demanding job in administration. Her hours were long and her stress was great, through work overload, whereas I, by contrast, was slipping into depression through the stress of loss (of school), loneliness and my inability to find anything to motivate me. When Anna returned home from a hard day at the computer, she wanted some space for herself, which was understandable. In practice, it meant a quick tea before diving up to her meditation room to check personal emails, watch her own TV and meditate—before an early night. So my day-time loneliness continued on into the evening. Weekends were better, with shopping trips to town, dances on a Saturday evening and, in better weather, Sunday afternoon gardening. But, weekends excepted, our drastically different work situations were pulling us apart.

4. As a result of my retirement, I suffered several losses—of intellectual enquiry, motivation and sociability with both staff and students. But I missed the interactions with the students most, as I saw and engaged with them more, through enquiry, debate and repartee. From the outset, I realised that my friendship with Jessie helped compensate for the loss of my student classes, and I missed them less thereafter (8.5). Then, during the long, lonely days with Anna out at work, Jessie's daily texts started to compensate—including my lonely evenings.

All this was epitomised by my 65th birthday, after Anna had flown off to India to be with her spiritual 'Master', leaving Jessie to provide me with company and support to celebrate my birthday in Anna's absence—for which I was grateful. Both Anna and I were in difficult, stressful places in our weekday worlds but, generally speaking, we didn't turn to each other for the support that we both needed. Anna was supported by her twice-daily meditation practices and by her Sunday morning meditation meetings and friends—and I was supported by Jessie. It is not surprising then that I became as attached to Jessie as Anna was to her meditation practices.

*

I did not mention my friendship with Jessie to Anna, naively thinking they could co-exist without coming into conflict. When Anna discovered our texting and dance friendship, this was no longer possible and conflict ensued. Consequently, there were many tortured conversations and post-dance inquisitions between Anna and myself. Clearly, Anna wanted me to detach myself from Jessie—but that was something I could not do, for Jessie's friendship was filling a large and important emotional space following my post-retirement losses and, increasingly, the space created by the growing distance between Anna and myself.

Therefore, Anna's request for a divorce, when it came, was no surprise to me, for it had already been mooted in our many conversations and arguments. So I was prepared—as I'd been seeking greater independence within the marriage for some time, of which *Café Pop* was a symbolic expression (8.5). I also took my problems with Anna and Jessie to Nancy's therapy room, where she helped me come to terms with what was going on. My long-standing friend Katie attempted to help Anna and I resolve our differences—but to no avail. We both appreciated her efforts on our behalf but our issues seemed unresolvable, at least within the marriage itself.

*

In the end, we divorced in 2016 but continued to live together in the marital home, largely without acrimony, until it was sold. We used the financial settlements to buy ourselves two very different properties only half a mile apart, as we both wanted to keep in touch. We are probably more supportive of each other now—especially during the pandemic—than we were in the latter part of our marriage. At Christmas, following our move, Anna sent me a card containing the following words:

You are not just my ex-partner, but still my supporter, my cheerleader, confidante and friend. I'm lucky to have you on my side and in my corner.

Our marriage had come to the end of the line—but our friendship, it seems, is coming around again.

9. Still Passionate!

2017–9

"Nancy, it's 2017 and I'm 67. It's just another year, and I'm drifting. Nothing is going to happen, so what's the point?"

"What's brought this on?" Nancy enquired. "The last time we spoke, you were fine."

"Just the January blues, I expect. Might have something to do with my divorce—and that I'm going to be on my own again. Oh, and Coventry City are going to get relegated again—down to where they were before I started supporting them!"

"You may find that your move to your new apartment works out better than you think. But I can't do much about your football team—I'm a therapist, not a magician."

*

So I'm back in Nancy's therapy room. Creative psychology has taken a backseat whilst Anna and I are preparing our home to be ready for sale and have started to divide up its contents. We're not fighting, but it's not a bundle of fun either. In March, we receive a definite offer.

Meanwhile, what had completely slipped my mind between my visits to Nancy and trying to sell the house, was that Coventry City were still in a minor cup competition. Two days after my 'January blues' session, they won a quarter-final on penalties and, by virtue of previous results, they would play their semi-final tie at home! Unfortunately, City hadn't won a League match for three months, so I had no expectations of semi-final success. It would be no contest and although the match was live on SKY, I'd be watching it from behind the sofa, like the horror film I was expecting it to be.

However, much to my amazement, the *Sky Blues* play really well, score two goals early on and end up 2-1 winners! It's scarcely believable, but in the midst of a terrible season, Coventry City are going back to Wembley—30 years after winning the F. A. Cup in 1987 (4.3). I have to pinch myself to believe it—along with the 40,000 other City supporters who make their joyous way to Wembley for an April Cup Final in the sun.

I obtain tickets easily enough for myself and Terry—a former school colleague, with whom I still attend the occasional match. Once again, the *Sky Blues* are the underdogs—this time to Oxford United who are pushing for promotion and who have already given City a 4-1 thrashing in the League. Like the 1987 heroes, however, City, under the new management of Mark Robins, seem perfectly at home in the National Stadium and play positive attacking football. After 10 minutes, they are 1-0 up, then 2-0 and they eventually run out 2-1 winners to win the EFL Trophy. Sky blue and white covers the whole of one end of Wembley, reminiscent of scenes of 30 years previously, as fans celebrate this surprising achievement. That is, until a month later—when the team is relegated, as expected, into the bottom division of the English football league.

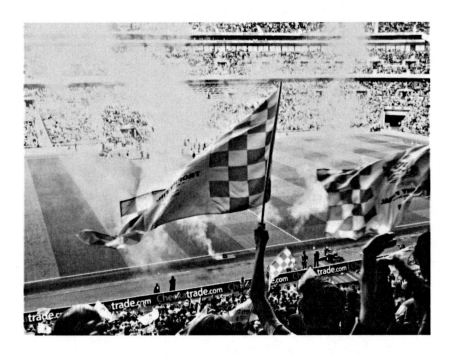

Back at Wembley again after 30 years—and to witness another victory.

347

The following season, with the manager making a host of new signings, hopes are high for a swift return to the division above, from whence they had just fallen. But the team is inconsistent and it's a rocky ride throughout the season, but the *Sky Blues*—with their tremendous 'away' support—keep within touching distance of the play-off places. Their form improves in the final few games, to get them into a semi-final play-off place against Notts County, a team local to where I'm now living.

After two incredibly tense games and with more than their fair share of luck, City end up as 5-2 winners over the two legs. It's difficult to believe, but the *Sky Blues* are back at Wembley for the second year running—for another Cup Final! On this occasion, City's opponents are Exeter City, who finished above City in the league. So officially, we continue to be the underdogs for our third Wembley final. But this time, with City's current excellent form, I'm confident of success. And I'm not disappointed as, after a goalless first half, City roar into a 3-0 lead after the break with some glorious goals—including full-back Jack Grimmer's curling left-foot shot that soars then dips—into the very top corner of the net! Once more, the *Sky Blue* song resounds around Wembley as the happy 40,000 City fans pay tribute to the new manager and his new-look team. This victory means that City are now promoted to the tier above—the club's first promotion since 1967! With Wembley success and now a promotion, the good times are coming around again for Coventry City—and hence for me!

Two months after the 2017 final, Anna and I move to our respective new homes: Anna to a semi-detached 3-bedroom house with garden and patio for her plants and pots. Myself to a modern 2-bedroom ground-floor apartment on a leafy estate. Katie helps me on moving day but after the dust settles, I know that there are a lot of improvements to be undertaken as soon as I can.

The most important of these for me is the recreation of *Café Pop* in my living room (8.5). Again, I have a stone-wall background upon which are displayed music memorabilia from my life in pop—with tributes to Bob Dylan, the Pet Shop Boys and Katy Perry, among many others. It reminds me of the decor at the Sun Studios Cafe in Memphis (8.3)—perhaps where I picked up the idea.

After a couple of months however, I realise that I've played no music at all at my new home despite all the CDs and vinyl that surround me. I'm missing the beat and feeling flat—but not for long as I spot *Lissie* [137] on a US TV show. I love her sound, her electric-acoustic guitar—and the beat! I buy two of her albums and enjoy air-playing my (miniature) Johnny Cash guitar to her songs. I tell Jessie about my discovery and ask her to watch Lissie on YouTube, which she does.

"Jamie, Lissie is very good, and if you like her, then you'll like Fleetwood Mac."

Of course, I'd heard of Fleetwood Mac but they had been formed in 1967, the year I gave up pop and got into evangelical religion, so I never got to know their music. So I borrow a CD from Jessie and I immediately recognise their hit songs, and love most of the rest. Music was back for me in my new apartment! But it didn't stop there, for once Jessie heard of my new-found enthusiasm:

"Jamie, there's a *Fleetwood Mac Tribute Band*—I'll look them up if you're interested."

So Jessie finds the *Rumours of Fleetwood Mac*—the tribute band that is officially authorised by Mick Fleetwood. They've finished their 2017 tour so Jessie books two tickets for their 2018 show in Nottingham. I'm blown away by their performance, especially the songs of Emily Gervers (aka Christine McVie) and Jess Harwood (aka Stevie Nicks). The next day, I snap up the last available seats at their Leicester, Lincoln and Sheffield concerts—as I still don't do things by halves. They always meet their fans after the show is over so they get used to seeing me! My favourite song is *Gypsy*—and in my musical pantheon, they are one of the *Seven Wonders* of the world!

*

Soon after moving into my apartment, I'm contacted by Fraser—an old friend from my time at St John's College, Durham. He had heard on the grapevine that I was living in the Nottingham area and took the trouble to look me up. He's still an Anglican minister belonging to a Nottingham parish and clearly doing a lot of good work, especially with refugees and asylum seekers. It's good to see him for a long catch-up! Afterwards, we arrange to meet every month or so, in Waterstones' Café. He has a wide cross-cultural and multi-disciplinary knowledge, so he is excellent to talk to and to discuss ideas with—

over cappuccinos and tea-cakes. My reconnection with Fraser has been a welcome and pleasant surprise and an opportunity to talk, enquire and debate once more—about worldwide migration and trafficking; the climate crisis; Brexit; Creative Psychology; mental health—and much more besides.

*

Jessie comes up with some surprises too—for in the month before my house-move, she had suggested that we might visit Rome for a long weekend to celebrate her birthday, which will be after my moving date. Never having been to Italy before and unsure about holidaying by myself, I take up her offer. It's a fascinating trip, especially seeing Raphael's *School of Athens* fresco for real in the Vatican, with Plato and Aristotle centre-stage—as distinct from seeing it on the front cover of every other philosophy textbook.

The following year, we undertake a similar weekend trip, this time to Florence and Pisa. All is going well until we step into our hotel room—where there is a double bed instead of the requested two singles. Jessie, horror-struck, flies down the stairs to reception to complain and order another room! Meanwhile, I'm upset by Jessie's insensitive reaction to the situation and upon her return, storm out of the room and into the narrow streets and rush-hour traffic of central Florence.

"I'm off—no idea when I'll be back!"

"Why? What for? Can I come with you?"

"No, you can't—work it out for yourself!"

Several hours later, I return to find two single beds and an apologetic Jessie. I'm also ready to apologise but keener to tell her what happened to me in Florence.

First, I call in at a nearby café to take a breath, calm down and enjoy some breakfast tea and a speciality cake. Outside again, I spy a major bookshop and discover an English section. After a while, I pull out a yellow-spined paperback—*The Pursuit of Happiness* by Ruth Whippman [138]. I had read a number of books on the popular 'happiness' theme, but this seemed different—and better. Not so much to do with the content and argument, but with the style. There are three aspects in particular that grab my attention:

1. It's a personal memoir about recent years spent in California, where the 'happiness' meme is big business!
2. It has narrative memoir and psychological understandings of 'happiness' running alongside each other; for me, a delicious combination of story and reflection.
3. It's written in the first person present—giving it dynamic and dramatic impact.

I'm hooked and can't put it down—until the lights are dimmed and we're given five minutes before the store shuts down for the day. Of course, I make the purchase before making my way back to the hotel and Jessie.

Later that night, wide awake in my single bed, I start to make a few connections. I had already made several attempts at writing my own memoir, but wasn't really satisfied with any of them—written as they were in the third person, past tense. But now I realise that perhaps I can do it differently—using the first person present and running a psychological analysis at the end of each chapter to keep story and reflection together—yet distinct. Over breakfast, I explain my ideas to Jessie and she is supportive, with some suggestions of her own. The remainder of our holiday is as much about my new inspiration as it is about leaning towers or statues of David.

Back in Nottingham, I put pen to paper, then keyboard to Word document, having devised eight chapters, each with its own psychological analysis of that chapter's storyline. Although inspired by Ruth Whippman's book, I had never seen anything like this arrangement before. I write furiously for six months—at which point it is more or less finished, and I am more or less satisfied. But what will others make of it?

My editor-in-chief, Katie, having improved my English no end, is very enthusiastic. And Curly, my long-standing friend, also thinks this is by far my best effort. But they are personal friends—can I get an external endorsement, even a publisher? After a few months, I get my answer in a Sunday evening email from Professor Jeremy Holmes, whose book about John Bowlby and Attachment Theory had crystallised my developing thoughts about attachment twenty-five years previously (4.9). He clearly likes it and among his other favourable comments is his opinion that it stands "head and shoulders above similar accounts". A few months later and my book is on the way to being published.

351

But I know next to nothing about publishing—so it's the start of a brand new journey for me—and who knows what possibilities and pitfalls lie ahead?

But for now, I have a new project and I'm more than happy to be passionate—about *'Passionate!'* [149A]

10. Retirement Crises: Review

i.   My mother's death and funeral (8.1) proved to be the trigger for a series of retirement crises, brought about by the coincidental timing of certain events and by the way in which Anna and I decided to use my share of her estate; i.e., our house purchase—the project that ended all projects. Spending a fortnight in close proximity to my brother Nigel was a unique but valued opportunity. Most people thought it extraordinary how such different characters could have the same parents. But I was aware that we also had our insecure attachments in common. Mine being anxious-ambivalent, with emotions bubbling away on the surface, with my brother clearly having an avoidant attachment, with emotion display being virtually non-existent. This, I can only assume, stemmed from a strict authoritarian and non-affectionate upbringing in the four years before I was born. My mother's 'Unforgettable Night' (1.1) doesn't appear to have affected Nigel in the way it affected me. With Nigel, it seems that the damage had already been done [139].

ii.   The trigger for my decision to retire at Christmas, rather than at the end of the academic year, was the increasing amount of work-related stress due to my losing control over the way in which I worked and taught (8.2). Or, as Ofsted might see it, my inability or unwillingness to adapt [140].

iii.   The overwhelming positive response I received from the students, both in their 'thank you' cards and also upon my dramatic later return, was due—in my view—to the positive, non-authoritarian and *interactive* way in which I taught. As attachment researchers soon came to realise, it is the *interactional* quality of parent-child relationships that is key to establishing secure attachments [141]. So it seems that, from the students' comments and sense of loss (and the 'abandonment issues' of some), there was a positive sense of bonding in the work we did together. My sixth-form work was therefore another institutional attachment for me, possibly triggered in 2004 by my adoption of a third 'A' level—the philosophy of religion: the same year that I married Anna.

iv.   My current employment in a local sixth form has helped mitigate this sense of institutional loss, as it provides my weeks with both structure and personal interactions. But the fact that it is a non-teaching role means that any interactions are more superficial and prosaic.

v.   Finally, I should add that the receipt of my retirement cards, from both students and staff, on my final day before Christmas was one of the most moving moments of my life—a positive affirmation of my sixth-form teaching career, Ofsted notwithstanding. In my pantheon of iconic moments, it almost ranks alongside Coventry City's 1987 Cup Final victory—but not quite!

vi.   The severe impact of my retirement didn't register at first as I had two new and exciting projects lined up: the search for a new house and location using the proceeds of my mother's estate. Also, the prospect of a fortnight's USA music tour with my grown-up godson, Ed (8.3). There was virtually no space in between the timings of these projects and no awareness of how retirement would affect me in the long term. It was a retirement 'honeymoon', which lasted for almost eighteen months before the dust finally settled. Such 'honeymoons' are characteristic of certain types of retirement but mine was rather unusual. For whereas a 'normal' honeymoon period might be enjoyed because of the delight of not working anymore, I was only too aware that, Ofsted apart, I really wanted to be back teaching again—*and in my way*, for that is what I enjoyed the most [142].

vii.   All honeymoons, however, come to an end, and the stark realities of retirement had to be faced, both external and internal. The realities were starker than I had imagined—for things had changed so much that they had left me 'a lonely man with an empty mind' (9.3).

viii.   My early post-honeymoon phase entirely justified those worries and fears. For, with the loss of sixth-form teaching and the honeymoon over, my life seemed denuded of the very core of my meaning and existence. Cycling around Rushcliffe Country Park in ever-decreasing circles (8.4) symbolised the futility of my post-retirement existence. It was some comfort to find such meaningless routines identified in Eliot's *I have measured out my life in coffee spoons*. But that didn't actually change anything in my situation and I was at a loss to know what would. I had not yet come to view my retirement as a 'career bereavement' (8.7), but according to attachment psychologists, I was suffering from 'chronic mourning', as had also occurred after Francesca had left (3.6)—years of unremitting grief, common to anxious-ambivalents [144].

ix.   My active (though futile) searching for meaningful activities was, in fact, a form of denial: I wanted a new attachment 'to make it all better'— a 'rebound attachment'—like a rebound relationship after a love affair ends. In both cases, it's to cover up the intense feelings of loss.

x.   In the second phase, my searching brought unexpected rewards, not in the form of a new attachment—but through revisiting scenes of unfinished business from the past; for example, my teenage rejection of both Subbuteo and my pop music collection. And, more poignantly, revisiting Durham—the site of my major trauma of faith—and the subsequent reframing of my Durham years as a crucible rather than a prison. In all these ways, I was investigating my 'shadow side' (Jung) and bringing it into the light. I was letting go of the need for quick-fix, fantasy attachments and addressing issues around my previous *real* attachments. In that sense, I was 'smelling the coffee', while, at the same time, in my external world, I was still measuring out my life with coffee spoons.

xi.   When I first met Jessie, her impact was considerable because her similarity to my sixth-form students meant that my chronic mourning for that institutional attachment was significantly reduced in its intensity. Due to my need to cling on to *something* from that institution, it is not surprising that she emerged as an attachment figure for me, substituting for the students themselves. Anna did not feel threatened by a school institution or by my commitment to it—but it's understandable that she felt threatened by Jessie, its attractive and very personable symbolic substitute.

xii.   In my period of clinical depression (8.6), it became clear that there were also age and identity issues present in my retirement scenario. Issues I could ignore for most of the time, but not on this occasion. However, 'The Black Hole' does illustrate that even with my 'shadow side' turning itself towards the light, and even with Anna present and Jessie becoming an attachment-figure, I *still* lacked a sense of meaning and purpose in retirement. This was central to my dilemma and remained so until the arrival of my Magic Moment and with it, Creative Psychology.

xiii.   My life-story has been punctuated by various 'Aha' moments (8.7), two of the most notable being my first visit to see Coventry City in 1959 (1.6) and then my reaction to the *McVicar* film (4.5) thirty years later. My Creative Psychology revelation fitted this pattern and was the most powerful and precise of them all. The Freud programme acted as a trigger, but the 'moment' came from within, not from without. There were underlying forces at work—most notably, Nancy's support of my creativity and Susan Cain's new psychology as seen in *Quiet*. New, that is, to me.

xiv.   There was also a less visible factor, namely that of my brain-circuitry. Claudia Kalb's article in a National Geographic magazine [145] proposed (on the basis of MRI scans of jazz musicians) that there are (at least) two different 'thinking' routes in our brain. Thinking that is driven, repeated and highly focussed occurs in the prefrontal cortex and is highly accessible to consciousness. But another route exists deep inside the mid-brain, of which we are normally less conscious: it is the route of less driven, but more imaginative, improvised and creative thought. It can't be tamed or regulated like the thinking in the prefrontal cortex. Kalb's article suggested that 'Aha' moments derive from the creative circuitry and therefore are, by definition, both creative and unexpected—but may be preceded by a period of contemplation—which I had been doing.

xv.   I had been teaching 'A' level psychology in highly driven and highly focussed and regulated ways for 15 years, along with two other 'A' levels. The details of the Specification Content were all-important. My prefrontal cortex would have been working in overdrive for all these years to deliver these courses—with my inner, creative circuitry hardly used, and certainly not in connection with psychology. Upon my retirement, I lost all interest in psychology. For teaching it in the way necessary to pass exams had slowly killed it for me. I now think that it took four years for my prefrontal cortex to quieten down and for my creative circuitry to be stirred up—by books such as Susan Cain's. With new, open-ended topics to contemplate and Nancy's affirmation of my creativity, Creative Psychology was born—the one single split-second moment that transformed my retirement.

xvi.   En route to this revelation, I was starting to accept my introversion that Cain's book had suggested. It made sense of many aspects of my life including my difficulties in various social situations, where I got quickly bored with chit-chat and often excused myself early with a sigh of relief. It also stopped me comparing myself negatively with people who had a 'full social life'.

xvii.   I simply didn't need it, realising that often, my best company was my own. As for my initial thought that the Introversion-Extroversion spectrum had little to do with Attachment Theory, this has been largely been borne out by research, the only exception being the strong correlation of those avoidantly attached with introversion [146]. But in general, attachment and personality appear to be two separate systems that interact with each other—rather than being predictive of each other.

xviii.   Our marital difficulties, it would seem, were largely down to me (8.8). My sexual disinterest in over-available partners is easily traceable to my infant experience of inconsistently available love. My preference for institutional attachments—such as Coventry City, evangelical religion and school teaching—stem from the same source, as they provided the *reliability* that, in my experience, most (but not all) personal attachments do not offer.

xix.   Therefore, it seems, in hindsight, that I was more strongly attached to my sixth-form teaching than I was to Anna—to my work more than to my marriage. Had Anna been less available, flirtier and flightier, then perhaps things might have been different—but that is pure speculation. In reality, Anna had no such character flaws. In theory, I could perhaps have resisted Jessie's offer of friendship, thus preventing my emotional attachment to her, but surely this would have just kicked the problems of my retirement into the long grass rather than solving them. They would surely have recurred further down the line.

xx.   Another cause of our marital problems was the 11-year age gap between us and the implications of that for when I retired: namely that our work trajectories were headed in opposite directions. At the time we married, my retirement was almost a decade away and we had no wish to speculate what the future might hold. So we both colluded in ignoring the issue.

xxi.   In my view (though not in Anna's view), the course of our marriage was subject to the social-psychological laws of the **fundamental attribution error**. This is: *a pervasive tendency to underestimate the importance of external situational pressures and to overestimate the importance of internal motives and dispositions in interpreting the behaviour of others.* [147] In other words, I think the best explanation for the collapse of our marriage is to be found in its circumstances: primarily my retirement and my prior attachment to my teaching role. But also the age gap between us, our different work trajectories and our different cultural backgrounds, including Anna's devotion to her meditation practices and to her spiritual Master.

xxii.   For Anna, the problems were not situational but dispositional—namely my willingness to allow 'three in the marriage'. I understand her viewpoint but again, I think she underestimates; surely not three but four or five—including my sixth-form work and her meditation as the other invited guests. But I do agree that, whether by virtue of situation or disposition, the marriage was indeed 'rather crowded'.

xxiii. The reason I chose a modern apartment for my new single life (8.9) was that I had realised by then that our lovely, semi-rural marital home was not for me. It was, as I sensed at the time, 'Dad's house'—a house and a location that he would have admired and loved. I think that was a choice by default for me as, at the point of search and purchase, I had no idea what I wanted to do with my retirement—so I was happy to experiment with something that was familiar, but new to me. I hoped it would provide Anna and myself with a new start for my retirement. It did—a bad start. Externally, picture-postcard beautiful. But inwardly, for me, isolating and alienating.

xxiv. At my new apartment, I have tree-lined streets and a large, well-maintained lawn—but maintained by others, not by me! I've no desire either to garden or cycle around country parks, even though there are fields and cycle paths nearby. I just need, and have, a warm, sunlit study where I can read and write and measure out my life with interesting books—as well as with the occasional coffee spoon.

xxv. External events have also impacted me very favourably in my short time here as a singleton. To see Coventry City play and win at Wembley is a wonder to behold, let alone twice in two years! I've also been fortunate to have discovered new upbeat music and go holidaying in Rome and Florence. And I can enjoy as much Test cricket and top football as I want via SKY—without having to justify it to anyone. I've also made new friends at dance and at my new school.

xxvi. Only two issues trouble me on a regular basis: when I go dancing, I still want to *talk* more than dance—a hangover, I suspect, of my chronic mourning for my sixth-form teaching. And I'm still unsure whether I'm independent enough to holiday by myself, but so far, I've not had to cross that particular bridge. But in the grand scheme of things, these are small inconveniences.

xxvii. What *has* surprised me however is how much I enjoy living by myself—in complete and total contrast to my life in Desolation Row [148]. For this, I have to thank good friends and therapists, fortuitous circumstances and a good deal of self-understanding. It may well be that alongside my ambivalent attachment, I have been able to build up some 'earned security', or what Jeremy Holmes refers to as *an internal secure base*, whereby an individual *feels more secure in himself* [149]. It certainly feels as though this is—or is becoming—the case.

xxviii.   To sum up: **Passions** are neither inherently positive nor negative. To be sure, I've experienced both the cataclysmic lows and unbelievable highs that passion brings in its wake. Left to its own devices, passion leaves us vulnerable. *It feels without seeing.* It is best accompanied by a strong dose of rational thought (4.6) to mitigate its excesses and extremes. Neither does passion originate exclusively in one's individual psychology. For passions can become ignited through group solidarity, such as in 'enthusiastic' religious gatherings or in political or protest movements with powerful agendas. From a moral viewpoint, passion can achieve great good or can take both individuals and societies into the depths of evil. Martin Luther King was passionate—yet so was Adolf Hitler. Passion without rational thought or moral guidance is indeed a dangerous emotion.

xxix.   To sum up: **Crises** come in all shapes and sizes, and we have all experienced at least one, by virtue of our birth. For most people, it will be more than one, and for some of us, many more. Of the various crises I've experienced so far, stretching over nearly seven decades, four stand out two negative and two positive:

Negative crises:

1. **My religious crisis**—because of its length and acute mental severity at the time. To not have 'God' in my life seemed at the time like the end of the world. But it wasn't.
2. **My retirement crisis**—because of its length and alienating affect. To not have teaching in my life seemed like not having a life at all. Today, I'm slowly building an enjoyable life without teaching—that's not to say that I don't still miss those sixth-form discussions and debates. I do.

3. Both religious and retirement crises were undoubtedly rendered more difficult and more prolonged by my anxious-ambivalent status: *chronic crises* as it were. However, understanding this brings relief and self-acceptance—so I don't beat myself up about it. It's who I am.

Positive crises:

1. **My Coventry City moment in 1987**—because of its external and surprising nature, and the depth of my re-attachment despite a 20-year absence. Moreover, because of its therapeutic effect in restoring a sense of post-religious identity and reconnection with my teenage self.
2. **My Creative Psychology moment of 2016**—because of its sudden, revelatory nature and the immediacy of its impact, banishing depression in a flash and transforming my retirement crisis from 'coffee spoons' to creativity—after a long and rocky road that broke my marriage with it.
3. For those with attachment difficulties like myself, there is a message loud and clear:
   Get to know and understand yourself as best as you can—through honest friends, therapy (where possible) and Attachment Theory as applied to yourself. Use this self-knowledge to be self-accepting—enabling you to 'hang in there' when times are tough. Then, when times are better, to enjoy your passionate life to the full!

*

To support positive mental health:

1. Early on in the chapter, the issue of *stress* arises—for both staff and students. Staff, as adults will have had prior experience upon which to base their dealing with it: *what's important, what's not so important, what are the options open to me?* Students, mainly because of their young age, will lack such experience. Therefore, it seems to me that it is beholden of the adults to *nuance* their expectations of students. Some students will rise to the challenge of high expectations and will feel fulfilled by that challenge. Many however will not and will suffer to the point of needing therapy or medication and may self-harm. Adults,

whether staff, parents or family friends, need to sense when a student is struggling and take some pressure off. *It's okay not to be an academic. It's okay not to meet your target grades. It's even okay to want a different sort of life.*

2. For most people, endings are also very difficult. Endings of holidays, endings of employment, endings of relationships. The ending of a life. But there is great diversity in this. For some, the ending of a particular employment (for example) is a massive relief to be celebrated! But for others, especially where strong bonds have been made, there is the need to mourn the loss. Positive mental health is best served in such circumstances *not* by 'looking on the bright side of life' but by appreciating what is gone, maintaining those links that will help preserve the memory and being willing to accept the sadness while it lasts. In all but the most extreme circumstances, it will pass—or at least be diminished. Like in the vast majority of mental health issues, there are positive ways forward to be sought out and worked on. But, apart from the occasional and unexpected 'Aha!' moment, there is rarely a quick fix. And even then, such joyous moments often only occur after extended periods of struggle, doubt or despair.

Conclusion ~ Towards Positive Mental Health

Conclusion

A. Four useful therapies

Depression, anxiety and an ambivalent sexuality have been the three mental health issues that I've had to contend with over the years. To help me cope with, and eventually resolve, these issues, I have been helped by four therapies—as described in greater detail in Chapter 4:

1. *Intensive psychotherapy*—following both religious and retirement crises. This provided me with a temporary secure base (the therapist) to help buffer the trauma and thus cope with everyday life better.
2. *Cognitive therapy*—from both therapist and wise friends who had 'both feet on the ground'. This helped me see things realistically and not fantastically, which is what I was prone to.
3. *Transactional Analysis*—to help me understand what was going on in various relationships, and how and why I responded to various people and events. Also, how I could make better choices—from my Adult.
4. *Attachment Theory*—to help make sense of diverse and chaotic experiences, and to help me understand how my past may have contributed to my later development and difficulties.

All of the above contributed significantly towards my improving mental health, with a minimal need for anti-depressants. Of course, many people will have more severe mental health problems than I have experienced and will require more specialist help and treatment. But any of the above four therapies provide a good starting point, if you are feeling mentally unwell and are in need of some help.

B. Attachment and positive mental health

1. *"Jamie, I think you will find that if you want to move forwards, you will first have to look backwards."* Those words from my therapist were not what I was wanting to hear. Nevertheless, thirty years later, I recognise that they are some of the most important words ever spoken to me, and one of the most important lessons I have learned in my 'passionate' journey. In our contemporary western culture, there are many voices urging us to live in the present—live for the moment—and almost as many promoting the future: 'moving on', 'going forward', 'where do you see yourself in ten years' time?' Fewer cultural voices are heard about regard for the past or, if so, only negatively: 'get over it!', 'stop living in the past'. Yet, if 'Passionate!' has taught me anything, it is that an awareness of one's own past is as essential for one's present and future mental health as a rear-view mirror is for keeping oneself safe on the road in order to pursue one's onward journey. It is always important for car drivers to know what lies behind them and what may be about to overtake them—from a speeding ambulance to a thunderous wagon rattling by, striving to meet company deadlines. Being overtaken by life-events is no less scary and this is only made worse if you are not expecting them or don't understand them. For example, I never expected that retirement would prove so very problematic to me, but at least I could understand it. *Attachment theory has thus become my rear-view mirror for daily living*—I need to keep checking what lies behind in order to remain safe in the present, while looking forward to what lies ahead. But Attachment theory has other important lessons too.

2. I have had to learn the hard way that attachments may be negative as well as positive. In itself, 'attachment' is a neutral term, simply describing a state of affairs, but the intensity and object of one's attachments may vary enormously and may have a variety of outcomes. In my own story, I can identify three such attachments that have severely troubled me, leading me at times to despair and, on one occasion, to foolishly risk my own life and the lives of others.

The first of these negative attachments was my insecure attachment to my parents. It was neither their fault nor mine when life-events overwhelmed us all (1.1), leaving the connections in my infant brain inadequately formed, resulting in subsequent emotional confusion and a desperate hunger for affection. Others, of course, have suffered far worse, such as outright rejection and infant abuse with their many varied and serious consequences: from a life in children's care homes to suicide—unless, of course, adequate therapeutic interventions are made through counselling and/or fostering, to help them uncover and deal with the ghosts of the past.

My second negative attachment (and an indirect consequence of the first) was my intense attachment to evangelical Christianity and all its works. Of course, there were positives, such as a new meaning and purpose in life and a source of social life and context for meeting girls. But eventually, my Biblical fundamentalism clashed with my emerging need for rational, evidence-based beliefs, and the five-year road of disintegrating faith was increasingly distressing, taking my meaning, identity, career and friendships into an abyss. However, I am not saying that all religious attachments (even evangelical attachments) necessarily have such damaging effects. For many people require some form of religious attachment as an existential necessity—especially in cultures or sub-cultures that are subject to ecological, geographical, economic or political insecurities. In such circumstances, religion may be the life-raft that keeps communities afloat and makes survival worth fighting for. For myself, however, my religious attachment proved to be negative—and *there are many other negative objects of attachment available* to those who feel emotionally or socially deprived, such as attachments to racial or nationalistic identities, to street gangs where parental care and control has gone missing—right through to the everyday attachments to smartphones and social media, the use of which for some borders on the obsessive. It's now commonplace to see an infant in its buggy being ignored by a parent on their smartphone—as opportunities are missed for those verbal and visual interactions that help build and maintain warm, loving and secure relationships.

My third negative attachment is more about the *intensity* of my emotions than the object of attachment itself. My early evangelical experience was emotionally intense as becoming 'one with Jesus' (i.e., merging with Jesus) was the desired goal. *But this 'merging' endangered my sense of identity* (even my life—as in 4.6) and it took me a decade or more to fully recover from this loss. Nevertheless, my potential for merging was clearly evident in my relationship with Penny, after which I needed help from Maggie once again. Merging one's identity with that of another person or institution may seem to the insecurely attached the means to a 'safe haven' of repose. But it comes at a very high price—namely the risk of feeing empty, distraught and lost when the other person pulls away or the institution is abandoned [150].

3. On my 'Passionate!' journey, I have also learnt that in order to undertake therapy, you have to be brave. My decision to see Maggie for help was one of the most difficult decisions I have ever made, despite the fact that it was borne out of utter desperation. A bit like going to the dentist for the first time after missing appointments for twenty years. It is certainly *not* like going to a café with a friend—therapy is no piece of cake. Just like at the dentist, you never know what the therapist may find, or what stories may need to be extracted before any remedial work can take place.

However you may think that, for a number of reasons, a visit to a therapist is just not for you. In which case, I suggest that you attempt the exercises in the Appendix as a means of self-therapy. The *Love Quiz* may give you some clues as to your attachment status and related issues. The *Ego-gram* may open your eyes to important aspects of your personality and your relationships with others. My mother often said to me: "You and me, we're always at cross-purposes—goodness knows why!"

I wanted to reply: "Because we have crossed transactions due to my being insecurely attached", but I never got around to that 'adult' conversation—perhaps I should have.

4. Perhaps the most obvious lesson I have learnt as I have explored my attachment-related issues is the distinction between attachments to people and attachments to institutions. This has only crystallised for me as a result of my retirement experience, viz my attachment to my specific form of educational work. John Bowlby once referred to '*our attachments to country, sovereign or church*' [151], but there seems to have been very little development of this theme in the volumes of attachment-related, post-Bowlby research. Kirkpatrick's work on religion is the obvious exception (see Ch. 2).

My present view is that *an attachment to an institution carries certain benefits, especially for the insecurely attached* who find trust in personal relationships problematic. An institution is less likely to personally reject an individual, and an institution has a feeling of permanence that personal relationships may not have. There is security in a big organisation and in big numbers. This chimes well with an emerging consensus in 'Happiness studies'

[152] that suggests that a major factor for individual happiness is *socialising with other people* [153]. And where does one find numbers of people socialising together? In institutions—in my case, on the terraces or stands with fellow Coventry City supporters; in the Church; on the dance-floor—and at work. But there's a snag.

What happens if the unexpected should occur and the institution you are attached to withers and dies? Or, more likely, *your interest withers and dies*? The fallout from either eventuality may be considerable. Not perhaps as sharp as the rejection by a friend or romantic partner, but very likely to be more all-encompassing. Institutions are more likely to define one's self-identity and role or roles in life. In my own case, I lost all sense of who I was after giving up my Anglican ministry and the Christian faith. It was a similar story when I retired from my teaching career. The sense of loss can resemble a tsunami—in that it removes all known landmarks, including existing personal relationships—as proved to be the case with me. It seems there is a need for a counterbalance—not exactly an early tsunami warning system, but at least a place to hide—a safe haven—when the giant waves strike.

5. In my experience, *the great counterbalance to both institutional and personal loss is an awareness of one's attachment history*—and one's style and propensity for attaching to this or that institution or person. To have this sense of understanding and ownership of one's life—what Jeremy Holmes calls 'autobiographical competence' [154]—gives one a sense of self that is not dependent upon other institutions or people. When my religious loss occurred, I had no understanding whatsoever of what was happening to me so I 'lost myself' in Francesca's love that, when withdrawn, led me into such desperation that I needed face-to-face therapy.

Retirement was different. To be sure, I was 'shell-shocked' when I realised how attached I had been to my school and sixth-form work, and how comprehensively its loss so denuded my life from both a social structure and a meaningful existence. But my awareness of my attachment history provided me with a framework for understanding what was going on—even if the actual experience was both long-lasting and very isolating. And in this sense, my retirement crisis was nothing like as devastating as my religious loss.

All this has confirmed the truth for me that *in order to move forwards, you may have to look backwards.*

Looking backwards while moving forwards may seem a tricky manoeuvre to pull off, but it's possible so long as we keep checking our rear-view mirror.

The mirror of attachment.

I believe that it's a major factor for developing and maintaining one's positive mental health—whether or not you are predisposed, like me, to live a passionate life.

Appendix: Two Personality Exercises

A. The Love Quiz

Introduction

The aim of this exercise is to help the reader identify their own attachment status. It may also raise other issues as well, concerning relationships with primary carers and romantic partners.

The quiz is based upon original research by Hazan & Shaver in 1987. It consists of 3 parts:

(a) self-description of early relationships
(b) self-identification with a 'romantic style'
(c) the matching of (a) and (b)

In classroom use, I found that about 75% of the students could match (a) and (b) and thus could clearly identify with an attachment status that they felt was accurate for them.

The quiz

(a) Self-description of early relationships.

Choose five adjectives that describe your relationship with your parents (or one of your parents) in your early years. Write them down in the spaces below.

1.
2.
3.
4.
5.

(b) Self-identification with a 'romantic style'

Read the three descriptors of romantic love, in X, Y and Z below. Place a tick next to the one that you think best represents how you normally feel in a romantic relationship. (If you identify with more than one descriptor, then you could prioritise them with a 1, 2, 3.)

X. I am somewhat uncomfortable being close to others; I find it difficult to trust them completely, difficult to allow myself to depend on them. I am nervous when anyone gets too close, and often partners want me to be more intimate than I feel comfortable with.

Y. I find it relatively easy to get close to others and I am comfortable depending on them and having them depend on me. I don't often worry about being abandoned or about someone getting too close to me.

Z. I find that others are reluctant to get as close to me as I would like. I often worry that my partner doesn't really love me or won't want to stay with me. I often want to merge completely with my partner, and this desire sometimes scares people away.

(c) The matching of (a) and (b)

(a) *If the majority of your adjectives in (a) are words like: cold, cool, distant, non-communicative, in awe of, etc.—this would signify an **avoidant attachment** to your parents (=AA).*

*If the majority of your adjectives in (a) are words like: warm, loving, close, kind, easy to talk to—this would signify a **secure attachment** to your parents (=SA).*

*If the majority of your adjectives in (a) are words like: confused, chaotic, anxious, unloved, angry, this would signify an **ambivalent** (anxious/resistant) **attachment** to your parents (=AMB).*

(b) *The romantic style descriptors:*
*X indicates an **avoidant** style (AA)*
*Y indicates a **secure** style (SA)*

Z indicates an **ambivalent** *style (AMB)*

Matching:

If your results are *two AA's*—this suggests an *avoidant attachment* with your parents, with a corresponding avoidant style in romantic relationships. This would seem to confirm your avoidant attachment status.

Two SA's would seem to confirm a *secure attachment*, both with your parents and in romantic relationships.

Two AMB's would indicate an *ambivalent (or anxious/resistant) attachment* with parents and romantic partners.

In many cases, there will not be a perfect matching up; in which case, other factors can be explored, such as gender influences and the attachment status/style of one's romantic partner. Attachment research seems to confirm that early childhood experiences will have a significant influence on later adult relationships,

For a fuller discussion of these issues, I commend: *Attached* by Levine & Heller. Rodale. 2010; for example, part three: *When Attachment Styles Clash.*

B. Ego-Gram

Introduction

The Ego-gram is to help ascertain the relative strength of various aspects of personality that are used in Transactional Analysis (4.2 in the main text). It is an aid to self-awareness. The ego-gram on page 377 was given to me in the therapy process, and I have used it successfully with many students. The vast majority came to recognise the results as accurate, after they were revealed.

1. Instructions

1. Next to each word, in each small box, place a + or a -, according to whether you normally use such a word, gesture, etc. in everyday life. If you normally do, put a +. If you normally don't, put a-. Fill in every small box in every column. E.g., if 'bad' is a word you don't often use in everyday conversation, then place a—in the small box in the top row for column 1. I have already done this for you—but if you do use the word 'bad' in normal conversation, then you can change this to a +. This is a quick-fire, gut-response quiz. You should take about 2 seconds for each small box and two minutes maximum for the lot.

2.When all the small boxes are filled with a + or -, then add up the plusses only, and write the total for each column in the appropriate space in the bottom row. ONLY COUNT THE PLUSSES. Ignore the minuses.

3 Then, on page 378, with a pencil, shade in the number of plusses (+) for each column, starting from 0 at the bottom and shading upwards until you reach the exact number. This will now give you a strong visual representation of key aspects of your personality that are important for your transactions/interactions with others.

	Col. 1	1	Col. 2	2	Col. 3	3	Col. 4	4	Col. 5	5
words spoken	bad	-	good		how?		I want		I can't	
	should		nice		what?		I won't		I wish	
	ought		poor thing		why?		here goes!		I try	
	must		I'll help		I think		ace!		I hope	
	always		don't worry		possible		hi!		please	
	ridiculous		never mind		probable		fun		thank you	
tone of voice used	telling off		loving		reasonable		loud		whining	
	ordering		comforting		enquiring		excited		grudging	
	disgusted		concerned		thoughtful		mischievous		willing to please	
gestures used	points finger		open arms		open		instant reaction		sulky face	
	frowns		hugs		calm face		flirty/sexy		sad face	
	angry face		smiling		alert		dramatic		innocent face	
attitudes displayed	fault finding		accepting		sensible		curious		accepting	
	right & wrong		understanding		logical		fun-loving		ashamed	
	bossy		empathetic		making sense		changeable		guilty	
Totals /15	+ for Col.1		+ for Col.2		+for Col.3		+for Col.4		+for Col.5	

	+ for Col. 1	+ for Col. 2	+ for Col. 3	+ for Col. 4	+ for Col. 5
15					
10					
5					
0					

Interpretation

Column 1 should give you an indication of your 'Critical Parent' strength.

Column 2 should give you an indication of your 'Caring/Nurturing Parent' strength.

Column 3 should give you an indication of your 'Adult/ rational' strength.

Column 4 should give you an indication of your 'Free Child' strength.

Column 5 should give you an indication of your 'Adaptive Parent' strength.

It is important to recognise that there is no 'perfect' or 'normal' pattern. It is the balance (or imbalance) of the various aspects that is important. For example, if you have a high score (10 or more) for your 'Caring Parent' (Column 2), then your kind nature might be taken advantage of—but this can be compensated for by a high score in your 'Adult' Column. If you have high scores for your 'Critical Parent' (Column 1) or 'Free Child' (Column 4), then you are more liable to have crossed transactions with other people. For further discussion on these and

378

related issues, look up Transactional Analysis/Ego-gram online or see the relevant section of Further Reading on page 393.

Notes

Desolation Row

1. *The Love Song of J. Alfred Prufrock.* Selected Poems, T. S. Eliot. Faber. 1961. For more on the influence of T. S. Eliot, see Ch.2.2.
2. ibid

1. Childhood Attachments

3. 1.6 *One Way Ticket.* Neil Sedaka. 1959. RCA. The 'B' side to *Oh! Carol.*
4. 1.8 *Eve of Destruction.* Barry McGuire. 1965. Dunhill/RCA.
5. 1.8 *The Times They Are A-Changin'.* Bob Dylan. 1963. Warner Bros. Inc.
6. 1.10 In current attachment literature, the terms *anxious attachment* or *resistant attachment* are often preferred to the somewhat ambiguous *ambivalent attachment.*
7. 1.10 *Probably [attachment] continues throughout life and, although in many ways transformed, underlies many of our attachments to country, sovereign or church.*
John Bowlby, 1956, cited in *Handbook of Attachment*, ed. J. Cassidy and P. Shaver (1999), The Guildford Press, p803.
8. 1.10 Although the strength of reaction and passion is characteristic of anxious/ambivalent attachment, the role of *inborn temperament* will also affect how strongly emotions are experienced, and behaviours presented, either modifying or exacerbating them.

2. Religious Crises

9. 2.1 the *Sky Blue Song:* written in 1962 by Coventry City manager Jimmy Hill, and club director John Camkin, for Coventry City supporters who have sung it at matches from 1962 to the present day.

9a. 2.1 *A Hard Day's Night.* The Beatles. E.M.I. Records Ltd. 1964.

10. 2.2 See Note 1.

11. 2.2 *The Waste Land.* Selected Poems, T. S. Eliot. Faber. 1961.

12. 2.2 Note 4 above.

13. 2.2 Dylan refers to T. S. Eliot in *Desolation Row* (1965), which some Dylan critics regard as his take on *The Waste Land.* Both Eliot and Dylan are recipients of the Nobel Prize for literature, Eliot in 1948 and Dylan in 2016.

14. 2.2 *The Hollow Men.* Selected Poems, T. S. Eliot. Faber. 1961.

15. 2.2 *Choruses from 'The Rock' II.* Selected Poems, T. S. Eliot. Faber. 1961.

16. 2.2 ibid

17. 2.2 *Choruses from 'The Rock' X.* Selected Poems, T. S. Eliot. Faber. 1961.

18. 2.2 ibid

19. 2.3 I Corinthians 1 v23

20. 2.3 RCA Victor/Decca Records 1967

21. 2.3 Romans 8 v28

22. 2.4 This event took place on 29 October 1968. For a docudrama reconstruction, see the film *McVicar* with Roger Daltrey and Adam Faith. 1980. The Who Films Ltd. For my delayed psychological response to these events, see Chapter 4.5.

23. 2.4 For the modern debate on this issue, see *The Self Illusion.* Bruce Hood, 2011, and *Freedom Regained.* Julian Baggini, 2015.

24. 2.4 1 Peter 4 v12-13

25. 2.5 For an insider's view of L'Abri, see *Crazy for God.* Frank Schaeffer, 2007.

26 2.5 Inter Varsity Press. 1968. 23C. Inter Varsity Press, 1969.

27. 2.5 ibid

28. 2.5 ibid

29. 2.5 Hans Rookmaaker. IVP. 1970.

30. 2.7 *Evil and a God of Love.* J. Hick, Fontana, 1977.

31. 2.7 Based on words by Karl Marx in the *Communist Manifesto*. Original 1848. His point was that mankind will at last face '*his real conditions of life*'. 1888 translation.

32. 2.8 Further publication by Fontana, 1976. According to the back cover, '*this shatteringly honest book...evokes a disturbing self-awareness in his reader.*'

33. 2.8 The themes death and resurrection are further developed in *The True Resurrection* by H. A. Williams (1972), Mitchell Beazley and 1983 Fount paperbacks.

34. 2.8 Extracts from the sermon *The True Wilderness*, p28-30.

35. 2.8 *Tensions*, Mitchell Beazley (1979) p28.

36. 2.9 *Sir Marcus Browning M.P.* from 'Rowan Atkinson, Live in Belfast' (1980).

37. 2.9 For a more recent example of turning away from faith with a great sense of loss, see *Unfollow* by Megan Phelps-Roper. Riverrun. 2019.

38. 2.10 Bowlby claimed that the initial two and a half years of a child's life was the critical period for the nature of a baby's attachment to be established, and this is supported by Sue Gerhardt: "that expectations of other people...are inscribed in the brain, outside of conscious awareness, in the period of infancy, and that they underpin our behaviour in relationships through life." *Why Love Matters*, Sue Gerhardt (2004).

Other studies and psychologists suggest a more flexible and lengthier 'sensitive period'.

39. 2.10 *Handbook of Attachment*. Cassidy & Shaver. The Guildford Press. 1999. p36.

40. 2.10 *Attachment in Adulthood.* Mikulincer & Shaver. 2007. p281.

41. 2.10 See the book of Revelation Ch.3 v20

42. 2.10 A summary of Kirkpatrick by Richard Gross in *Themes, Issues and Debates in Psychology*. R. Gross (2003) p177.

43. 2.10 St John's Gospel Ch.3 v16

44. 2.10 Marcia identifies four: Identity diffusion, Identity foreclosure, Moratorium and Identity achievement. See *Human Growth and Development*. Beckett & Taylor (2010) p98.

45. 2.10 See *Behave*. R. Sapolsky (2017) p154.

46. 2.10 ibid. p155.

47. 2.10 *Attachment, Evolution and the Psychology of Religion*. Lee A. Kirkpatrick (2005) p159, The Guildford Press.

48. 2.10 ibid p151

49. 2.10 *Secure base* and *safe haven* are two complementary functions of any attachment figure, the former generating confidence to be outward bound, and the latter providing care and protection as and when needed.

50. 2.10 This belief was always a childish fantasy, and its importance to me was a measure of my extreme neediness for assurance about the reliability of my divine attachment figure. A much more sensible and scholarly approach to the Bible can be found in *The Bible for Grown-Ups.* Simon Loveday (2016).

51. 2.10 see note 35. p137.

52. 2.10 ibid

53. 2.10 Erikson believed that individuals pass through eight psychosocial stages, each with its own 'crisis' (in a neutral sense) to deal with. If issues at one stage are not properly resolved, then one will have to revisit them at a later stage before one can move on.

3. Romantic Passions

54. 3.1 The Five Points of Calvinism were formulated at the Synod of Dort in the Netherlands (1618-19) as a critical response to The Five Articles of the Arminians. Though not used widely by Calvinists, they regained their popularity in the 20th century. A secular view would regard them as both highly immoral and socially divisive.

55. 3.2 'Do not be mis-mated with unbelievers': 2 Corinthians 6 v14.

56. 3.8 *Games People Play.* Eric Berne (1964) Penguin Random House (2016) p114-5. Eric Berne is the founding father of *Transactional Analysis:* see 4.2.

57. 3.8 *Women Who Love Too Much.* Robin Norwood (1986 and 2004) Arrow Books. Norwood's argument is that women who have this 'love-addiction' are suffering from a psychological problem similar to alcohol addiction that requires a similar recovery programme as is used by Alcoholics Anonymous.

58. 3.8 *Diana: Her True Story.* Andrew Morton (1992) Michael O'Mara Books. This is the first semi-autobiographical account of the problems that rocked the royal family and brought about the divorce between Princess Diana and Prince Charles. It would seem likely that Diana's upbringing and psychological troubles may well have influenced William and Harry in their promotion of charities that support psychological health and well-being.

59. 3.9 *John Bowlby & Attachment Theory.* Jeremy Holmes (1993) Routledge. The updated second edition, 2014, contains more recent research as well as a chapter on Attachment Theory and mental health.

60. 3.10 See 40 above, p58-61. Also, Sir Richard Bowlby, John Bowlby's son, cites his father referring to an attachment *pyramid*—with the principal attachment figure at the top, subsidiary figures underneath and friends and familiar neighbours forming the base. *Fifty Years of Attachment Theory.* Sir Richard Bowlby (2004) Karnac Books Ltd.

61. 3.10 See Note 39 above, p14.

62. 3.10 See Note 59 above. 2nd edition, p20. This account is supported by John Bowlby's son, Sir Richard Bowlby, who suggests that the trauma of this loss for his father was in fact the motivation for his research and work on the attachment bond.

63. 3.10 Mary Ainsworth, a student under John Bowlby, became a collaborator with him on Attachment Theory, devising 'The Strange Situation' research method to analyse the different types of attachments. She became a leading child psychologist in her own right.

64. 3.10 There is no suggestion that the continuity from attachment *types* to romantic *styles* is automatic or genetic. Overall, the research on 'the continuity hypothesis' suggests that about 25-30% of people change their attachment type as they proceed from childhood to adulthood. Secure attachment may be *earned* (see 3.10 *iv*) or, in adverse circumstances, it may be lost. The style of a partner may be a contributing factor for change.

65. 3.10 *The Psychology of Relationships.* Julia Willerton (2010) Palgrave MacMillan. p53.

66. 3.10 See Note 59 above. 2nd edition, p168.

67. 3.10 This is an issue that returned and was of greater consequence in later relationships (5.6 and 7.7). See *Mating in Captivity.* Esther Perel (2007) Hodder.

68. 3.10 Avoidant/avoidant pairings probably hold the worst prospects for successful relationships as in: *How Psychology Works.* ed. J. Hemmings (2018) DK Penguin Random House, p157.

69. 3.10 ibid: for a near perfect summary of our ambivalent/ambivalent [anxious/anxious] coupling.

70. 3.10 See the excellent *Love Sick* by Frank Tallis (2004), which suggests that falling in love is akin to suffering an episode of mental illness. Arrow Books.

4. Therapies

71. 4.2 See note 56 above. *Parent, Adult and Child* are Berne's updated form of Freud's *Superego, Ego and Id*—but with the focus on behaviour rather than the unconscious.

72. 4.3 *Coming Around Again.* Carly Simon. Arista label. UK release January 1987—charted at no. 10. Provided the soundtrack for the film, *Heartburn.*

73. 4.3 St. Luke's Gospel Ch.15 v11-32

74. 4.3 *The Sky Blue Song.* Words by director John Camkin and manager Jimmy Hill (1962). Sung to the tune of the Eton Boating Song.

75. 4.4 Cyrille Regis MBE, centre forward for West Bromwich Albion, Coventry City, Aston Villa and England. Awarded the MBE in 2008 for services to charity and football. He died in January 2018 aged 59. A sad loss to both family and football at such an early age.

76. 4.5 *McVicar.* The Who films. 1980.

77. 4.6 *The Cognitive triad* proposed by Aaron Beck in 1976 as part of a cognitive-therapeutic understanding of depression. The terms used in this section are widely available in books and on courses of cognitive therapy, e.g., *10 Steps to Positive Living.* Windy Dryden (2014) (2nd edition) Sheldon Press, based on Rational-Emotive Therapy.

78. 4.7 See *TA Today. A New Introduction to Transactional Analysis.* I. Stewart, V. Joins (1987) p103. Second Edition 2012 available.

79. 4.8 *Lipstick on Your Collar.* Connie Francis (1959) Polydor Ltd.

80. 4.8 *Lipstick on Your Collar.* Dennis Potter (1993) Channel 4.

81. 4.8 *When All Is Said And Done.* Abba (1981) Polar Music.

82. 4.9 'The Strange Situation' experiment consists of a number of young mothers and their nine-month-old children in a controlled setting with concealed cameras and a one-way mirror. Up to nine very short 'situations' take place, including, for example, a mother leaving the room without her child and being replaced by a 'strange' mother-figure. The reactions of the child are observed, recorded and classified. This methodology is deemed both reliable and valid, and used worldwide, with overall consistent results.

83. 4.9 *Are Mothers Really Necessary?* 1987. Repeated on ITV Yorkshire in 1993.

84. 4.9 In the film, and also in *Attachment and Loss* Vol.1. J. Bowlby (1969) Pimlico ed. 1997 pxi.

85. 4.9 *Maternal deprivation* was the issue Bowlby focussed on before arriving at Attachment Theory. By it, he meant a child's physical loss of its mother (or mother-substitute) through either a long- or short-term separation, or through death. Later, he came to see that maternal deprivation could also be emotional as well as physical, through neglect, inconsistent care or purely a lack of affection and love.

86. 4.9 *John Bowlby and Attachment Theory*. Jeremy Holmes (1993) Routledge. Second ed. 2014.

87. 4.9 For romantic styles, see 3.10 *iii*. Also see Appendix A: The Love Quiz (Hazan & Shaver).

88. 4.10 Cited in Jeremy Holmes, see 86 above. Second edition, p134.

89. 4.10 ibid p137

90. 4.10 This is not meant to detract in any way from the therapist's role in healing through talking. It is more a distinction between primary and secondary roles in the healing process.

91. 4.10 Although, as I write, even the very existence of the club is far from certain, as SISU—the current owners—seem ambivalent about the future location of the club's base, which potentially could risk the club's future in the football league.

92. 4.10 The securely attached will not normally develop psychological problems. The avoidantly attached will normally reject any need for introspection due to the underlying pain and/or trauma that is responsible for their avoidance.

93. 4.10 *Maternal Deprivation Reassessed*. M. Rutter (1981) Penguin.
The Development of the Person /The Minnesota Study. L.A. Sroufe, et al (2005) The Guildford Press.

94. 4.10 See note 83.

5. Emerging Passions

95. 5.2 *Elementary Forms of the Religious Life*. E. Durkheim (1912)

96. 5.2 The prime example that Weber cites for his theory is *The Protestant Ethic and the Spirit of Capitalism*. Max Weber (1905). In his view, it was the Protestant Ethic of thrift that initiated and then maintained the capitalist enterprise of Western Europe and the USA.

97. 5.2 *The Managed Heart*. A. R. Hochschild (1983) California Press. *The Presentation of Self in Everyday Life*. E. Goffman (1959) Penguin ed. 1969. Hochschild argues that service workers (e.g., cabin crew) are routinely expected to present positive emotions in their work, resulting in many losing their own sense of identity. She draws upon Goffman's ground-breaking book, and her own research, to help justify her claims.

98. 5.3 I learnt a few years later that one of the senior staff who had undertaken training in TA had become head teacher in a neighbouring school and had introduced TA to Year 7, with the effect that behavioural issues were significantly reduced.

99. 5.9 Evangelicals discount *reason* as a means to establish God's existence, as it has been corrupted by original sin. Instead, they place all trust in God's revelation through an infallible Bible, which presumably has not been affected by sin, original or otherwise.

100. 5.9 The *Cosmological* argument is that the universe must have been caused by Something. The *Teleological*—that the universe suggests purpose, and hence an intelligent Designer. The *Ontological*—because, if God is Perfect, he must exist because to exist is more perfect than not existing. All these arguments are still debated vigorously by both sides, although the majority of philosophers reject any claims of their proof of God's existence.

101. 5.9 *The God Delusion*. Richard Dawkins. Originally the Bantam Press, 2006.

102. 5.9 For String Theory, i.e., the basic sub-atomic building block, my initial reading was: *Parallel Worlds*. Michio Kaku (2006) Penguin, Ch.7 & 8. Also: *The Goldilocks Enigma*. Paul Davies (2006) London.

103. 5.9 *Sacred and Secular*. P. Norris & R. Inglehart (2004) Cambridge University Press. This is the best and most comprehensive account I have read about the state of religion in the world.

104. 5.10 For 'merging', see 4.6

105. 5.10 These themes originate from Erving Goffman's influential work: *The Presentation of Self in Everyday Life*. 1959. Penguin ed. 1969. See also A. Hochschild, note 91 above.

106. 5.10 The reason that my internal, self-directed critical parent didn't show up on the Ego-gram is because TA is primarily concerned with outward actions rather than the inner workings of the mind.

107. 5.10 A story that most students of sociology come across at some time and which never fails to amuse can be found in a report by Taylor & Walton, entitled *Industrial Sabotage: Motives & Meanings* (1971). 'They had to throw away half a mile of Blackpool rock last year, for, instead of the customary motif running through its length, it carried the terse injunction 'FUCK OFF'. A worker dismissed by the sweet factory had effectively demonstrated his annoyance by sabotaging the product of his labour.' Anthony Ward, Cheadle Hulme, Cheshire.
108. 5.10 See Note 47 above, p106.

6. Mid-Life Crises

109. 6.1 See Note 58 above.
110. 6.2 *Jack Vettriano*. Text by Anthony Quinn (2004) Pavilion books.
111. 6.7 Icon books: a wide-ranging series of paperbacks covering many aspects of philosophy and culture. The text is lavish with cartoon illustrations that make them very accessible and a cheap, quick read.
112. 6.8 *Put On Your White Sombrero*. An excellent but lesser known ABBA song. Recorded in 1980 but only released in 1994, failing to make the *Super Trouper* album. Polar Music.
113. 6.8 With apologies to any female readers from Hull or Grimsby. This quip is based purely on negative regional stereotypes and is not based on any social research, so far as I am aware.
114. 6.9 *Castles in the Sky*. Ian Van Dahl. May 2000. No.1 in Scotland and in UK dance charts.
115. 6.9 Virtually a direct quote from *Acts 16 v31*. She had been taught well.
116. 6.10 Of course, if my substitute attachments should 'die': Coventry City through mismanagement (a distinct possibility at the time of writing), or dance through ill-health or disability, then they will be mourned too—though not in the same way, as they lack the sharp focus of a personal attachment figure.
117. 6.10 Individuation: according to Jung, it is the process whereby an individual learns to look beyond their focussed, 'one-sided' personality, to wake up to other, deeper aspects of themselves, such as their 'shadow' side, their creative side or their opposite-sex side.
118. 6.10 See *Human Growth and Development*. Beckett & Taylor (2010) Sage, p123.

119. 6.10 *Max Weber: Politics and the Spirit of Tragedy*. J. P. Diggins (1996) Basic Books. p63-5 and 297-8.

120. 6.10 *Sociology* 7th ed. A. Giddens and P.W. Sutton (2013) Polity Press. p352.

121. 6.10 *Lifespan Development* 2nd ed. Helen Bee. Longman. p408. Bee is a severe critic of the concept of a mid-life crisis, but allows this exception, based on Tamir's 1982 research.

122. 6.10 See note 40 above Ch.7 *Attachment Processes and Emotion Regulation.* esp. p203-4.

7. Russian Revolution

123. 7.9 *Stephen Fry in America*. Harper Collins (2008)

124. 7.10 See Note 63. 'The Strange Situation' procedure is one of the most common to be carried out in child psychology research for the past fifty years, with consistent results worldwide.

125. 7.10 *Attachment in Adulthood.* see note 40. p356

126. 7.10 *Mating in Captivity*. E. Perel (2007) Hodder. p107. Perel's book refers to a variety of reasons why some people suddenly lose sexual interest in their partner.

127. 7.10 ibid. p109.

128. 7.10 *The Chemistry of Connection*. S. Kuchinskas (2009) New Harbinger Publications Inc. p22.

8. Retirement Crises

129. 8.3 *Things Have Changed*. Bob Dylan. Special Rider Music. 1999.

130. 8.3 The opening lines, now adapted to my situation.

131. 8.4 See Note 1.

132. 8.4 *A Companion to T. S. Eliot*. Ed. David E. Chinitz (2009) Wiley-Blackwell.

133. 8.5 Attributed to Fran Drescher.

134. 8.7 *Retirement: the Psychology of Re-invention*. K.S. Shultz ed. DK Penguin Random House. 2016. p36-7 et al.

135. 8.7 *Quiet*. Susan Cain (2012) Penguin. Her sources include the *Myer-Briggs personality test*, which is itself rooted in the thinking and works of Carl Jung.

136. 8.7 University of the Third Age. After giving up on the table tennis, I joined the Psychology group.

137. 8.9 *Lissie*. American singer-songwriter. b.1982. *My Wild West* was the featured song.

138. 8.9 *The Pursuit of Happiness*. Ruth Whippman (2016) Winmill Books.

139. 8.10 The ITV character *Doc Martin* is clearly portrayed as being avoidantly attached, and he himself admits to an attachment order diagnosis in a counselling session. His parents are also portrayed as persistently rejecting him from the day he was born. Martin Clunes plays the title role.

140. 8.10 Professor Marmot's *Whitehall Civil Servant* studies show, among other things, that lack of control over one's work can have a negative impact on levels of both mental and physical health.

141. 8.10 Known as sensitive responsiveness and/or interactional synchrony.

142. 8.10 See note 134 p96-7 and 130-1.

143. 8.10 See note 131.

144. 8.10 See note 39 above, p736ff. Research suggests that those ambivalently attached are, in particular, prone to experience 'chronic mourning'.

145. 8.10 National Geographic, May 2017. p43-4. Claudia Kalb.

146. 8.10 See note 40 above p260-2.

147. 8.10 *Oxford Dictionary of Psychology*. Andrew M. Colman (2009) 3rd ed., Oxford University Press.

148. 8.10 For how single life can be enjoyable, I commend: *The Unexpected Joy of being Single*. Catherine Gray (2018) Aster. Moreover, the author commends Attachment theory for making the most illuminating sense about relationship psychology, p180-1.

149. 8.10 See note 86 above. 2nd ed. p137.

149A And within a few months of this conclusion, I had yet more to be 'Passionate' about—as Coventry City became Champions of Division 1 in the pandemic-reduced season of 2019-20. This, in turn triggered my first book: 'Attached to Coventry City—a personal memoir'. Pitch Publishing. 2021.

Conclusion

150. For this term and discussion, see *Attachment in Psychotherapy*. David. J. Wallin (2007) The Guildford Press. p225.

151. *Handbook of Attachment*. Cassidy & Shaver (1999) The Guildford Press. p803.

152. For example, in *The Pursuit of Happiness*. Ruth Whippman. See note 138.

153. Whippman rather belatedly adds that: *the single biggest factor affecting our long-term happiness and success is the love and warmth of our mothers.* ibid p261.

154. *John Bowlby and Attachment Theory*. Jeremy Holmes (2014) Routledge. p135.

In the same paragraph Holmes refers to an "autobiographical narrative" which *creates out of fragmentary experience an unbroken line or thread, linking the present with the past and future. Narrative gives a person a sense of ownership of their past and their life.*

Further Reading

Introductions to Psychology and Sociology

Butler-Bowdon, T. (2007) *50 Psychology Classics*, Nicholas Brearley Publishing.

Giddens, A. and Sutton, P. (2013) *Sociology 7th ed*, Polity Press.

Grenville-Cleave, B. (2016) *Positive Psychology*, Icon books.

Harvey, A. and Puccio, D. (2016) *Sex, Likes and Social Media,* Vermilion.

Jarrett, C. (2011) *The Rough Guide to Psychology*, Rough Guides/Penguin.

Mann, S. (2016) *Psychology*, Teach Yourself/John Murray Learning.

Osborne, R. and Van Loon, B. (1999) *Sociology*, Icon books.

Rooney, A. (2019) *Think like a Psychologist*, Arcturus Publishing Limited.

Seager, P. (2014) *Social Psychology*, Teach Yourself/John Murray Learning.

Snowden, R. (2006) *Freud*, Teach Yourself/Hodder Education.

Snowden, R. (2006) *Jung*, Teach Yourself/Hodder Education.

Ward, G. (2003) *Postmodernism*, Teach Yourself/Hodder Education.

Webb, R. et al. (2016) *AQA Sociology*, Napier Press.

Attachment and the Life-Course

Adams J. (2021) *Attached to Coventry City.* Pitch publishing

Beckett, C. and Taylor, H. (eds.) (2010) *Human Growth & Development*, Sage.

Bee, H. (eds.) (2011) *Lifespan Development*, Longman.

Bowlby, J. (1997) *Attachment & Loss. Vols.1-3*, Pimlico edition.

Bowlby, J. (2005) *The Making & Breaking of Affectional Bonds*, Routledge Classics.

Bowlby, J. (2005) *A Secure Base*, Routledge Classics.

Bowlby, R. (2004) *Fifty Years of Attachment Theory*, Karnac.

Cassidy, J. and Shaver, P. (1999) *Handbook of Attachment*, Guildford Press.

Cavendish, C. (2019) *Extra Time*, Harper Collins Publishers.

Gerhardt, S. (2004) *Why Love Matters*, Routledge.

Gross, R. (2003) *Themes, Issues & Debates in Psychology. Ch.9*, Hodder & Stoughton.

Harris, D. L. (ed.) (2011) *Counting Our Losses*, Routledge.

Holmes, J. & Slade, A (2018) Attachment in Therapeutic Practice. Sage.

Holmes, J. (eds.) (2014) *John Bowlby and Attachment Theory*, Routledge.

James, O. (2002) *They F*** You Up*, Bloomsbury.

Kuchinskas, S. (2009) *The Chemistry of Connection*, New Harbinger Publications.

Linsey, P. (1996) *Lifespan Journey*, Hodder & Stoughton.

Maddox, L. (2018) *Blueprint*, Robinson/Little, Brown Book Group.

Mikulincer, M. and Shaver, P. (2007) *Attachment in Adulthood*, The Guildford Press.

Milne, D. (2004) *Coping with a Mid-Life Crisis*, Sheldon Press.

Rutter, M. (eds.) (1981) *Maternal Deprivation Reassessed*, London: Penguin.

Sapolsky, R. (2017) *Behave*, Vintage books.

Shultz, K. S. (ed.) (2016) *Retirement: the Psychology of Reinvention*, DK Penguin Random House.

Sroufe, L., et al. (2005) *The Development of the Person*, The Guildford Press.

Timpson, J. (eds.) (2018) *A Guide to Attachment*, Timpson Ltd.

Transactional Analysis

Berne, E. *Games People Play*, Penguin: 1966. Penguin Life (ed.) 2016.

Harris, T. (1967) *I'm Ok—You're OK*, Arrow Books.

Lapworth, P. and Sills, C. (2011) *An Introduction to Transactional Analysis*, Sage.

Stewart, I. and Joines, V. (2012) *TA Today*, Lifespace Publishing.

Romantic Relationships

Ansari, A. (2016) *Modern Romance*, Penguin.

Bexker-Phelps, L. (2016) *Love: the Psychology of Attraction*, DK. Penguin.

Bradshaw, J. (2014) *Post-Romantic Stress Disorder*, Piatkus.

Dawson, J. (2017) The Gender Room. Two Roads.

De Botton, A. (2012) *How to Think More About Sex*, MacMillan.

Fisher, H. (2016) *Anatomy of Love*, W. W. Norton & Company.

Fromm, E. (1995) *The Art of Loving*, Thorsons/Harper-Collins.

Gottman, J. (1997) *Why Marriages Succeed or Fail*, Bloomsbury.

Gray, C. (2018) *The Unexpected Joy of Being Single*, Aster.

Jenkins, C. (2017) *What Love Is*, Basic Books.

Jones, W. (2016) *The Sex Lives of English Women*, Serpent's Tail.

Karter, J. (2012) *Psychology of Relationships—a practical guide*, Icon Books.

Levine, A. and Heller, R. (2010) *Attached*, Rodale.

Marshall, A. (2016) *I Love You But I'm Not In Love With You*, Bloomsbury.

Norwood, R. (1986) *Women Who Love Too Much*, Arrow books/Random House.

Perel, E. (2007) *Mating in Captivity*, Hodder.

Perel, E. (2019) *The State of Affairs*, Yellow Kite/Hodder.

Persuad, R. (2006) *Simply Irresistible*, Bantam Books.

Sternberg, R. (1998) *Love Is A Story*, Oxford University Press.

Tallis, F. (2005) *Lovesick*, Arrow Books/Random House.

Tallis, F. (2018) *The Incurable Romantic*, Little, Brown.

Templar, R. (2016) *The Rules of Love*, Pearson.

Willerton, J. (2010) *The Psychology of Relationships*, Palgrave MacMillan.

The Psychology and Sociology of Religion

Argyle, M. (2000) *Psychology and Religion*, Routledge.

Hinde, R. (2010) *Why Gods Persist*, Routledge, Taylor & Francis Group.

James, W. (1902) *The Varieties of Religious Experience*, Oxford University Press. (ed. Bradley, M. 2012)

Kirkpatrick, L. (2005) *Attachment, Evolution & the Psychology of Religion*, The Guildford Press.

Norris, P. and Inglehart, R. (2004) *Sacred and Secular*, Cambridge University Press.

Lowenthal, K. (2000) *The Psychology of Religion*, One World Oxford.

Loveday, Simon (2016) The Bible for Grown-Ups. Icon Books.

Phelps-Roper, M. (2019) *Unfollow*, Riverrun.

Sacks, J. (2015) *Not in God's Name*, Hodder & Stoughton.

Sargant, W. (1997) *Battle for the Mind*, Malor Books.

Williams, H. A. (1965) *The True Wilderness*, Collins Fount Paperbacks.

Williams, H. A. (1976) *Tensions*, Mitchell Beazley Publishers Ltd.

The Self

Bastian B. (2019) *The Other Side of Happiness.* Penguin Books

Burnett, D. (2016) *The Idiot Brain*, Guardian books and Faber & Faber.

Burnett, D. (2018) *The Happy Brain*, Guardian Faber.

Cain, S. (2013) *Quiet*, Penguin Books.

Critchlow, H. (2019) *The Science of Fate*, Hodder & Stoughton.

Dolan P. (2015) *Happiness by Design.* Penguin Books.

Goffman, E. (1971) *The Presentation of Self in Everyday Life*, Pelican/Penguin.

Haidt. J. (2006) *The Happiness Hypothesis.* Arrow Books.

Harris S. (2012) *Free Will.* Free Press

Hochschild, A. (1983) *The Managed Heart*, University of California Press.

Hood, B. (2011) *The Self Illusion*, Constable.

Klinenberg E. (2014) *Going Solo.* Duckworth Overlook.

Lawton, G. and Webb, J. (2017) *How to be Human*, New Scientist/John Murray.

Malkin, C. (2015) *The Narcissist Test*, Thorsons.

Nettle, D. (2007) *Personality*, Oxford University Press.

Precht, R. (2011) *Who Am I?*, Constable.

Stephens, R. (2015) *The Black Sheep*, John Murray Learning.

Trivers, R. (2013) *Deceit & Self-deception*, Penguin.

Verhaeghe, P. (2014) *What About Me?*, Scribe.

Whippman R. (2016) *The Pursuit of Happiness.* Windmill Books

Therapy and Self-Help

Briers, S. (2012) *Psychobabble*, Pearson Education Limited.

Butler-Bowden, T. (2017) *50 Self-help Classics*, Nicholas Brearley Publishing.

Clare, A. *In the Psychiatrist's Chair*, Vol.1, Heinemann 1992. Vol. 2, Mandarin 1996. Vol. 3, Catto & Windus 1998.

Dryden, W. (1994) *10 Steps to Positive Living*, Sheldon Press.

Dryden, W. and Gordon, J. (1990) *What is Rational-Emotive Therapy?*, Gale Centre Pub.

Foulkes, Lucy (2021) Losing Our Minds. Bodley Head

Grosz, S. (2013) *The Examined Life*, Chatto & Windus.

Holmes, J. (2001) *The Search for the Secure Base*, Brunner-Routledge.

James, O. (2010) *Britain on the Couch*, Vermilion.

Jenner, P. (2008) *Living Longer, Living Well*, Teach Yourself/Hodder Education.

Joseph, A. (2016) *Cognitive Behaviour Therapy 2nd ed.*, Capstone.

Kashan, T. and Biswas-Diener, R. (2015) *The Power of Negative Emotion*, Oneworld Pub.

Olson, D. (2017) *Success: the Psychology of Achievement*, DK. Penguin Random House.

Orbach, S. (2018) *In Therapy*, Profile Books.

Persuad, R. (2007) *The Mind*, Bantam Press.

Thorne, B. (1992) *Carl Rogers*, Sage Publications.

Tomley, S. (2017) *What Would Freud Do?*, Cassell/Octopus.

Wallin, D. (2007) *Attachment in Psychotherapy*, The Guildford Press.

Ward, I. and Zarate, O. (2011) *Psychoanalysis: A Graphic Guide*, Icon Books.

Yalom, I. (1991) *Love's Executioner & Other Tales of Psychotherapy*, Penguin.